Wissenschaft und Technik stellen zentrale, aber paradoxe Antriebs-
kräfte gesellschaftlicher Veränderung dar. Gesellschaften sind elementar
auf diese angewiesen, ihr Beitrag ist zugleich oft umstritten. Die Reihe
Wissenschafts- und Technikforschung eröffnet ein Forum, um diese
Entwicklungen insbesondere aus der Perspektive von Soziologie, Philo-
sophie, Sozialanthropologie und Geschichtswissenschaft auszuleuchten,
und bietet wissenschaftliches Grundlagen- wie wissenspolitisches
Orientierungswissen.

Schriftenreihe
„Wissenschafts- und Technikforschung"
NEUE FOLGE

herausgegeben von

Prof. Dr. Stefan Böschen, RWTH Aachen

Prof. Dr. Gabriele Gramelsberger, RWTH Aachen

Prof. Dr. Jörg Niewöhner, HU Berlin

Prof. Dr. Heike Weber, TU Berlin

Bis einschließlich Band 18 herausgegeben von:

Prof. Dr. Alfons Bora, Universität Bielefeld

Prof. Dr. Sabine Maasen, TU München

Prof. Dr. Carsten Reinhardt, Universität Bielefeld

PD Dr. Peter Wehling, Universität Frankfurt am Main

Band 22

Phillip H. Roth

Medicine as Science

The Making of Disciplinary Identity
from Scientific Medicine to Biomedicine

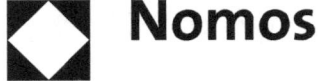 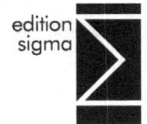

The Deutsche Nationalbibliothek lists this publication in the
Deutsche Nationalbibliografie; detailed bibliographic data
are available on the Internet at http://dnb.d-nb.de

a.t.: Bonn, Univ., Diss., 2021

ISBN   978-3-8487-8750-0 (Print)
         978-3-7489-3188-1 (ePDF)

British Library Cataloguing-in-Publication Data
A catalogue record for this book is available from the British Library.

ISBN   978-3-8487-8750-0 (Print)
         978-3-7489-3188-1 (ePDF)

Library of Congress Cataloging-in-Publication Data
Roth, Phillip H.
Medicine as Science
The Making of Disciplinary Identity from Scientific Medicine to Biomedicine
Phillip H. Roth
226 pp.
Includes bibliographic references.

ISBN   978-3-8487-8750-0 (Print)
         978-3-7489-3188-1 (ePDF)

1st Edition 2022
© Phillip H. Roth

Published by
Nomos Verlagsgesellschaft mbH & Co. KG
Waldseestraße 3–5 | 76530 Baden-Baden
www.nomos.de

Production of the printed version:
Nomos Verlagsgesellschaft mbH & Co. KG
Waldseestraße 3–5 | 76530 Baden-Baden

ISBN   978-3-8487-8750-0 (Print)
ISBN   978-3-7489-3188-1 (ePDF)
DOI   https://doi.org/10.5771/9783748931881

Onlineversion
Nomos eLibrary

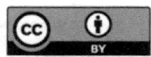

In memory of Reuben E. DeLoach

(1941–2016)

Table of Contents

List of Abbreviations

AEC	United States Atomic Energy Commission
APS	American Physiological Society
EBM	Evidence-Based Medicine
NASA	National Aeronautics and Space Administration
NIH	Institutes of Health (United States)
NSF	National Science Foundation (United States)
OSRD	Office of Scientific Research and Development (United States)
SSK	(The) Sociology of Scientific Knowledge
STS	Science and Technology Studies
TR	Translational Research
R&D	Research & Development
RCT	Randomized Controlled (Clinical) Trial

Acknowledgements

This book is a revised version of my doctoral dissertation in sociology, submitted to the Faculty of Philosophy at the University of Bonn in December 2020. Writing the thesis and the book has been like a journey for me – both intellectually and geographically. I would not have come this far without the generous help of many lovely colleagues, friends and family.

My project began to take on its current shape after I approached David Kaldewey at his group's summer school "Science and Politics" in September 2018 at the Forum Internationale Wissenschaft (FIW) in Bonn. Because of him, I was able to turn my inchoate ideas about science, medicine and politics into a challenging sociological research question about the institutional and conceptual history of the biomedical discipline. I owe him my sincere gratitude for his genuine interest in the project, for agreeing to supervise it and for continually pointing me in the directions most fruitful for pursuing my problem. I also gained a lot from Désirée Schauz and her work on the historical semantics of science in Germany and the USA. Not only did she act as the second supervisor to my thesis, but I also thank her cordially for encouraging me to strengthen the historiographical aspects of my book as well as for critically reading the final manuscript. Having such keen and benevolent supervisors was truly a blessing. But I need to also express gratitude to the other members of my doctoral committee, chair Clemens Albrecht and examiner Rudolf Stichweh, who made my defense a pleasant and memorable event despite the restrictions due to the coronavirus pandemic.

Although not originally conceived in this context, I find it more than fitting that my book was finalized and published while working at a center for advanced studies in the philosophy, sociology and history of science and technology devoted to the theme of "research cultures". I am very happy to have landed at the Käte Hamburger Kolleg: Cultures of Research (c:o/re) for new and exciting intellectual adventures! I am especially indebted to our directors Gabriele Gramelsberger and Stefan Böschen, who as editors of *Wissenschafts- und Technikforschung* at Nomos offered to publish my book in the series. Stefan Böschen also deserves extra special thanks for the more than generous support that allowed making this an open access-book.

I'm delighted to thank many different people scattered throughout the country, who helped and supported me at different times during my journey towards a doctoral degree. In early 2016, I was fellow in residence at the Kolleg Friedrich Nietzsche in Weimar, where I first began to endeavor into the social study of biomedicine. I therefore thank its former director Rüdiger Schmidt-Grépály for granting me an opportunity of deep and "free-spirited" engagement that reoriented my professional trajectory to social theory and the relationships between biopolitics and modern health care institutions. I must also mention Werner Stegmaier in gratitude. Though we never discussed any of the topics in my book, he taught me to think with Nietzsche and Luhmann in a way that also radiates throughout the text.

I had the opportunity to present portions of my project at different occasions, for which I am grateful. I want to thank my interlocutors at the self-organized doctoral colloquium at the University of Duisburg-Essen in Summer 2018 for their comments on early ideas. Moreover, Helene Gerhards, Florian Rosenthal, Seçkin Söylemez, Alex Struwe and Stefan Vennmann were my academic companions in Duisburg during some of the crucial years of my doctoral studies and therefore deserve my heartfelt gratitude. Thanks are also due to the attendees of the research colloquium at the FIW in Bonn in January 2019. I also received valuable feedback from the participants of Mariacarla Gadebusch Bondio's Medical Humanities "Science Lab" in spring 2020, especially from Tommaso Bruni, Christian Kaiser and Emilia Lehmann. Shout-outs also go to Julia Schubert, who became one of my "best academic companions" while I was enrolled as a doctoral student at the university of Bonn. My colleagues at c:o/re in Aachen, too, deserve special mention: Ana María Guzmán Olmos, Stefanie Haupt, Dawid Kasprowicz and Alin Olteanu read parts of the manuscript and gave very useful comments for improving the text.

There are no words that can express the gratitude I feel for my parents, Susan and Jens Roth. They have supported me with great patience and sincerity in my – arguably precarious – career choice. This book is for you! My siblings Noreen, Justin and Sean never doubted my capabilities for becoming an academic (the only one in the family), even in moments of great setbacks; and I never want to miss the delighting and refreshing diversions you've offered me throughout my time working on this project. But I owe my greatest debt to my wife Franka: she has patiently and constantly offered support and guidance in many forms. She's been there from day one of my journey on the rocky paths of academia. The immense joy and unconditional love that she and our two daughters, Rosa and Rubina, bring to my life, are what keeps me going in a world currently lined with crises and disaster. For our two girls, I hope I can do my humble part to leave this place a little better than I found it.

1. Introduction: Science and Medicine – Two Cultures Lost in Translation?

In 2008, science reporter Declan Butler published a piece in *Nature* about the current state of biomedicine titled "Crossing the Valley of Death". The article talks about how in recent decades there has been a growing concern that the vast expenditures in biomedical research no longer add up to the expected health care returns. While researchers have made "huge strides [...] in understanding disease mechanisms", these have not resulted "in commensurate gains in new treatments, diagnostics and prevention" (Butler 2008: 840). The main reason for this crisis in biomedical productivity seems clear: "Over the past 30 or so years, the ecosystems of basic and clinical research have diverged" (ibid.). Put differently, there has been a growing tension between the cultures of laboratory science and clinic medicine. As agencies for medical research across the globe "are experiencing a similar awakening" (ibid.), they are making efforts to solve the problem of the ruptured relationship between the two cultures.

The article goes on to explain how the National Institutes of Health (NIH) in the United States, under the auspices of Elias Zerhouni, a radiologist and director of the NIH since 2002, designed a new vision of biomedicine to confront the troubles in the system. Zerhouni and the NIH consulted with "over 300 of the nation's biomedical leaders from academia, government, and the private sector" (Zerhouni 2003: 63) about the challenges facing biomedical research in the twenty-first century. In 2003, Zerhouni announced "The NIH Roadmap", a trans-institutional conceptual framework to be launched the following year, which resulted in the sweeping reorganization of the agency's institutional and operational structures as well as its funding schemes (Zerhouni 2003). A signature feature of "The NIH Roadmap", as Butler notes, is the attempt at "bridge-building" between basic science and clinical medicine (Butler 2008: 840). In this context, the concept of translational research, which has since also developed into a key component of the biomedical enterprise as such, has played an important role. Translational research (sometimes alternatively called "translational science" or "translational medicine") is a broad term comprising different organizational concepts for transforming knowledge from basic research into tangible clinical approaches (van der Laan/Boenink 2015, Blümel et al. 2015). With "The NIH Roadmap", the agency fostered the establishment of a network of translational research "hubs" and launched the Clinical and Translational Science Awards to encourage close collaboration between scientists and clinicians amongst others.[1]

However, Butler's *Nature* article is not only important as a contemporary testimony on biomedicine. It also showcases an iconic depiction of the cleavage between the cultures of basic research in the lab and patient care in the clinic. The image, which is meant to illustrate the biomedical situation and the need for translational efforts "between bench and bedside", is valuable because it provides a deeper look at the somewhat conflicting understandings of biomedicine that exist today. The image features the cartoon of two figures standing on opposing edges, connected merely by a rundown and rather untrustworthy rope bridge (figure 1.1.). Between them is the eponymous "valley of death", the "chasm" that "has opened up between biomedical researchers and the patients who need their discoveries" (Butler 2008: 840). The figure on the left represents the lab researcher; on the right side is the clinician. Both appear to be looking at each other in doubt. As the researcher puts one foot out to check the bridge's suspension, both are questioning whether it is a safe passage to deliver his/her message across to the clinician, who appears to be treating a patient with an unhappy expression on his/her face. At the bottom of the valley of death, in the middle, is a human skeleton; a stark reminder that "neither basic researchers, busy with discoveries, nor physicians, busy with patients, are keen to venture there" (ibid.). So, where is the conflict in this depiction of biomedicine?

---

1 https://ncats.nih.gov/ctsa/about (accessed March 9, 2022).

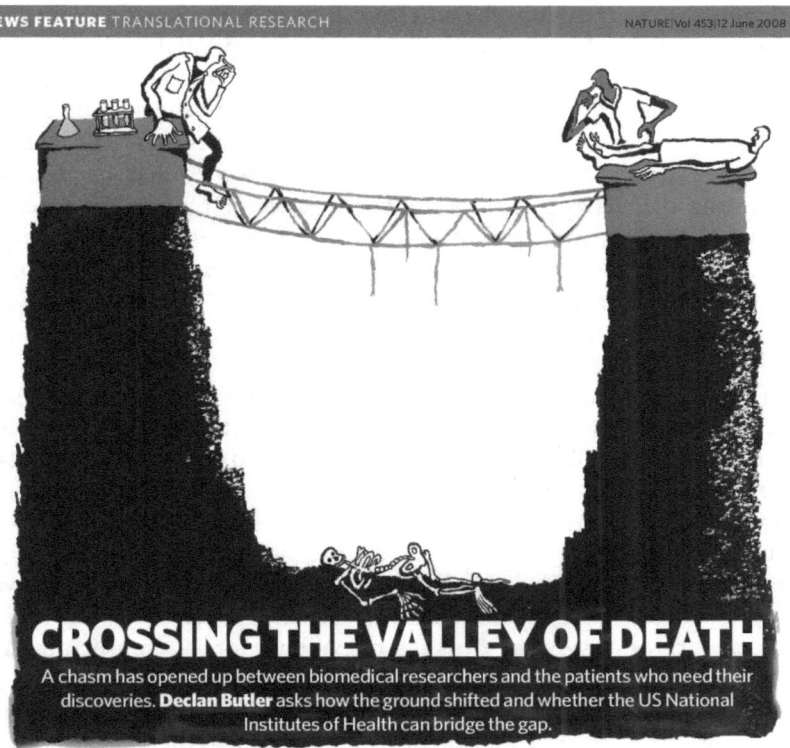

NEWS FEATURE TRANSLATIONAL RESEARCH   NATURE|Vol 453|12 June 2008

CROSSING THE VALLEY OF DEATH

A chasm has opened up between biomedical researchers and the patients who need their discoveries. **Declan Butler** asks how the ground shifted and whether the US National Institutes of Health can bridge the gap.

"NIH stands for the National Institutes of Health, not the National Institutes of Biomedical Research, or the National Institutes of Basic Biomedical Research." This jab, by molecular biologist Alan Schechter at the NIH, is a pointed one. The organization was formally established in the United States more than half a century ago to serve the nation's public health, and its mission now is to pursue fundamental knowledge and apply it "to reduce the burdens of illness and disability." So when employees at the agency have to check their name tag, some soul searching must be taking place.

There is no question that the NIH excels in basic research. What researchers such as Schechter are asking is whether it has neglected the mandate to apply that knowledge. Outside the agency too there is a growing perception that the enormous resources being put into biomedical research, and the huge strides made in understanding disease mechanisms, are not resulting in commensurate gains in new treatments, diagnostics and prevention.

"We are not seeing the breakthrough therapies that people can rightly expect," says Schechter, head of molecular biology and genetics at the National Institute of Diabetes and Digestive and Kidney Diseases in Bethesda, Maryland.

Medical-research agencies worldwide are experiencing a similar awakening. Over the past 30 or so years, the ecosystems of basic and clinical research have diverged. The pharmaceutical industry, which for many years was expected to carry discoveries across the divide, is now hard pushed to do so. The abyss left behind is sometimes labelled the 'valley of death' — and neither basic researchers, busy with discoveries, nor physicians, busy with patients, are keen to venture there. "The clinical and basic scientists don't really communicate," says Barbara Alving, director of the NIH's National Center for Research Resources in Bethesda.

Alving is a key part in the NIH's attempt to bridge the gap with 'translational research'. Director Elias Zerhouni made this bridge-building a focus in his signature 'roadmap' for the agency, announced in 2003 (see *Nature* 425, 438; 2003). Spearheading the NIH effort will be a consortium of 60 Clinical and Translational Science Centers (CTSCs) at universities and medical centres across the country, which will share some US$500 million annually when they are all in operation by 2012. Late last month, the NIH doled out the most recent grants in

B. MELLOR

Figure 1.1: First page of Declan Butler's article in Nature with a depiction of the "valley of death" in biomedicine. (Source: Declan Butler. 2008. Translational Research: Crossing the Valley of Death. Nature 453 https://www.nature.com/articles/453840a [accessed March 9, 2022]).

Upon closer inspection, the article with its imagery is ambivalent about what constitutes the normal and what the exceptional relationship between laboratory research and clinical care – an impression that nicely sums up general lines of argument in the literature. On the one hand, it presents the exceptional state of the successful connection of science and clinical practice across the divide as the norm – something, which derives from what I in chapter 6 call the *linear legacy* of biomedicine, i.e., the culmination of scientific expectations in the conviction that "laboratory research on basic biological mechanisms in almost any organism has potential medical relevance" (Scheffler/Strasser 2015: 664). On the other hand, the picture is clearly dominated by the considerable cleavage between the two cultures, something that appears as "natural" or literally set in (mountain) stone. Stated differently, the idea of mending the gap with the help of translational research implies a "broken middle" in the biomedical system (Mittra 2016: 57). This is indicated by the belied expectations in health care returns, which point to problems with the transmission of basic research results to clinical practice. And since this problem has supposedly only occurred recently, there is an inclination to accept that the normal state of biomedicine must be that of a harmonious relationship between the two cultures; one where – to keep with the imagery – a steel-enforced concrete bridge, instead of a rugged one, allows for a smooth connection between the lab and the clinic.

Much of the sociological and historical literature on the topic gives off this impression. Here, a crucial pier of that supposedly sturdy bridge is seen to have emerged through molecular biology. In their pathbreaking book *Biomedical Platforms*, for instance, historian Peter Keating and sociologist Alberto Cambrosio argue that "since World War II, biology and medicine have come together both institutionally and intellectually, in a hybrid practice that is neither syncretic nor synthetic" (Keating/Cambrosio 2003: 1, see also 330f.). Their study is a major contribution to the history and sociology of biomedicine, serving as the authoritative source on the topic for many other authors (e.g., Bruchhausen 2011, Crabu 2018, Löwy 2011, Qurike/Gaudillière 2008 Scheffler/Strasser 2015, Strasser 2014). The main reason for this new level of communication between the laboratory and the clinic is taken to lie especially in the "molecularization" of biology and medicine (Chadarevian/Kamminga 1998), which has allowed both cultures to become aligned with each other, i.e., to communicate with each other through "entities and tools" that are intelligible to both (Keating/Cambrosio 2004). In this part of the literature, biomedicine is consequently portrayed as coinciding "with the appearance of a new system of medical innovation in relation to biology and health policy" (Quirke/ Gaudillierè 2008: 445). Its central promise is that basic biological research will eventually lead to significant improvements in health care.

However, the image of a bridge connecting the peak of science to that of the clinic – whether stable or volatile – rather indicates that it is the divide between the cultures of science and medicine itself that constitutes the normal condition. The relationship between basic laboratory research and clinical practice is far more contested and precarious from this perspective. In this relation, the *Nature* article gives a different story of the molecular turn in biology and medicine. Butler explains that "basic and clinical research were fairly tightly linked in agencies such as the NIH" in the 1950s and 1960s. But with the "explosion of molecular biology in the 1970s", basic and clinical research have been separating, "and biomedical research emerged as a discipline in its own right, with its own training" (Butler 2008: 841). This left the enterprise in short supply of clinician-scientists, those medical professionals understood as straddling research at the lab bench and patient care at the bedside, who have become closely linked to the idea of translational research (Hendriks/Simons/Reinhart 2019).

Looking at the problem historically, the precarious image of the relation between science and medicine becomes dominant. As historian Steve Sturdy has noted: "One recurring theme" in the historical literature on science and medicine "has been to highlight instances of tension and conflict between medical science and clinical practice, or between medical scientists and clinical practitioners" (Sturdy 2011: 739). A central question therefore is why our society has today grown accustomed to the harmonious image, in which biology and clinical medicine are closely connected, instead of to the picture of a cultural divide. I will show that this has much to do with the history behind the narrative provided by biomedicine's *linear legacy*.

When medical research began to become professionalized in the nineteenth and early-twentieth century, though, the cultures of laboratory science and clinical practice were still largely distinct. Discrepancies (and even animosity) governed the relationship between the practicing physician and the laboratory researcher during that time, as studies in the social history of science and medicine have shown (e.g., Geison 1979, Lawrence 1985, Maulitz 1979, Warner 1991, 1992). In the post-Civil War United States, for instance, the appearance of the laboratory was initially perceived as a threat to the professional identity of the medical practitioner, who defined himself through the interaction with patients, and not through a devotion to scientific study (Warner 1986, 1992, see also Geison 1979). Keating and Cambrosio (2004) furthermore argue that eminent figures, such as the French physiologist Claude Bernard or the German pathologist Rudolf Virchow, who attempted to bridge the disparate scientific and clinical cultures, nevertheless retained an experimental and institutional division. Even those actors mentioned by Butler, who emerged in the early-twentieth century and who were socialized in natural science as well as clinical care, distinguished their research culture of clinical science – as I will show later in chapter 7 – clearly from that of the medical lab researcher, who dominated medical schools and research institutes (Kohler 1982: 221).

I. Towards a Historical Sociology of Medicine's Disciplinary Identity

How, then, can the idea of biomedicine as a hybrid of biological research and clinical practice be reconciled with the notion of an institutional and practical division between science and medicine? How has the exceptional state of bridging basic research and health care turned into our normal and deep-seated expectation of biomedicine, concealing the considerable divisions between lab and clinic? What are the consequences of this popular narrative for the organization of science and medicine as academic institutions and practices? And what did the public, politicians or society more generally expect of science in medicine and health care in the past?

This book tries to give answers to these questions by examining the changing understandings of science's role for medicine since the emergence of the modern research university circa 1800. It aims to show how our society's expectations of science and medicine have evolved and how they have shaped the social, cultural and epistemic constitution of academic medicine. For this purpose, I will trace the development of medical science as a modern institution from nineteenth-century Germany through to the rise of biomedicine in the postwar USA and to its current state at the start of the twenty-first century. Rather than working out the peculiarities of a given period, therefore, my study uses a long timescale that will allow to integrate specific historical phenomena into a general idea of the long-term developments of academic medicine[2] (Pickstone 2000: 5f.). This will help focusing on the tensions between change and continuity inherent to the modern history of medical science. Science seems to have been important for medicine throughout modernity. But how have research

---

2 I use the terms "academic medicine" and "medical science" interchangeably here.

practices and the ideas about their utility for medical purposes changed over time?

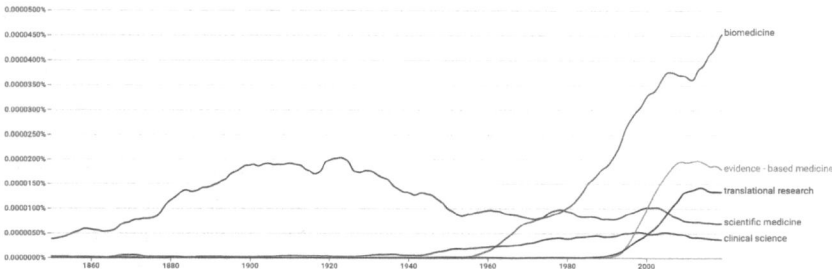

Figure 1.2: *Word frequencies of key medical concepts, 1850–2010. (Source: Google Books Ngram Viewer* https://books.google.com/ngrams/graph?content=scientif ic+medicine%2Cbiomedicine%2Cclinical+science%2Cevidence-based+ medicine%2Ctranslational+research&year_start=1850&year_end=2010 &corpus=26&smoothing=3&direct_url=t1%3B%2Cscientific%20medi cine%3B.t1%3B%2Cbiomedicine%3B%2Cc0%3B.t1%3B%2 Cclinical%20science%3B%2Cc0%3B.t1%3B%2Cevidence%20-%20base d%20medicine%3B%2Cc0%3B.t1%3B%2Ctranslational%20research%3 B%2Cc0 [accessed March 9, 2022]).*

My investigation takes on the form of a historical sociology of medical science. But I will not be telling a linear story. The aim is rather to highlight crucial episodes and to reconstruct important events in the institutional development of medicine as an academic science and in the organization of medical research. I will be focusing on professional trajectories and organizational programs that have significantly shaped academic medicine in the nineteenth and twentieth century. Germany and the USA are my national foci. Both countries were in their own ways and at different times in history crucial for the development of medical science, as I will show.[3] I argue that these developments can only be understood properly if academic medicine is observed in terms of a genuine scientific discipline. The historical and sociological literature on science and medicine, however, has

---

3 Michel Foucault's (1976) pioneering work on the medical gaze, in contrast, has put France in the spotlight for the development of modern medicine. However, Foucault emphasizes how especially the science of pathological anatomy enabled a conception of modern clinical practice. My concern is more broadly with the overall idea of medical science.

largely overlooked the *disciplinary* identity of medicine. Instead, medicine is treated mostly as a profession, connected to the university only through the academic training of physicians; and science features here mainly as an emblem of professional authority, rather than as a pursuit of its own (e.g., Starr 1982). Medical scientists, in turn, are viewed as "generally inclined to pursue their own independent research programmes", separated from clinical medicine (Sturdy 2011: 744). Consequently, the history of medical science has been told mainly as a pre-history to the history of biology and the biosciences (e.g., Zammito 2018). What precisely is meant by disciplines and disciplinary identity will be explained in the next chapter.

A possible reason why medicine's disciplinary identity has remained obscure in the literature is because the academic discipline of medical science – in contrast to other disciplines like biology, chemistry or physics – did not always go by the same name.[4] In fact, I will show how the designation has changed significantly. The most prominent semantic shift is that from "scientific medicine" in the nineteenth and early-twentieth to "biomedicine" in the second half of the last century, but also others have emerged over time, like clinical science or evidence-based medicine (figure 1.2). I will demonstrate the importance these different concepts have had to reformulating the disciplinary identity of medical science. To reveal the history of medicine as the social history of an academic discipline thus constitutes a necessary, albeit neglected, task of the social study of science.

The changing names for academic medicine from roughly 1800 until today provide an access point to the social history of medical science as a discipline and organize my investigation accordingly. They point to intellectual, professional and institutional programs through which actors tried to ensure the formation, growth and maintenance of an academic discipline of medicine in its own right, with its own research and training. I am interested in how these heterogeneous and conflicting programs have over time contributed to the formation of medicine's disciplinary identity. I thereby try to go beyond more traditional ideas of disciplines as the formal organization of scientific activity and scholarly education compartmentalized into university departments or institutes, or as institutions defined by special intellectual paradigms and practices (Roth 2022). Instead, my analysis employs an understanding of disciplines as products of cultural activity (Gieryn 1995, 1999, Lenoir 1997, Schweber 2006, Shapin 1992). Following sociologist Thomas Gieryn, they can be viewed as nothing "but a [cultural]

---

4 The term "biology", for example, appeared in 1800 and has since denoted the academic field (Nyhart 1995, Zammito 2018).

space". He argues that "Science is a kind of spatial 'marker' for cognitive authority, empty *until* its insides get filled and its borders drawn amidst context-bound negotiations over who and what is 'scientific'" (Gieryn 1995: 405, see also 1999: 18ff.). And it is within this space that Gieryn sees boundary work abound, i.e., discursive demarcations about what defines science in contradistinction to other cultural activities (Gieryn 1999: 12).

Another, complementary way of putting it, is to conceive of science as comprising a "supercategory". With linguist Roy Harris these function "to integrate what would otherwise be separate activities and inquiries; and the result of that integration is to re-draw the map of the intellectual world that society as a whole adopts" (Harris 2005: xi).[5] Taken together, what belongs to medicine as a scientific discipline happens through acts of symbolic integration and demarcation; through repeated discursive negotiations over what types of practices, actors, institutions, concepts, instruments and other elements are granted or denied authority over academic issues of disease, life and health – i.e., the cultural space of "medical science". And it just as much includes the ideologies, ideals, desires and expectations attached to these elements and to science and medicine as a whole. This moves my investigation away from concerns with specific scientific practices or theories to the realm of their cultural representations. However, a supercategory does not necessarily need to denote a specific discipline. As will become clear when I discuss the concept of biomedicine in later chapters, it can also act as a label that groups heterogeneous practices, research cultures and scientific epistemologies together in a manner that they conflict with each other and with established disciplinary identities. The result, as I will show, is an ambiguous notion of what a vast enterprise like medical science is expected to deliver to society.

Libby Schweber (2006) offers a good example of examining the institutional history of disciplines through the frame of "cultural space" in her comparative historical sociology of demography and vital statistics in nineteenth-century England and France. She emphasizes her study as one concerned with disciplinary *activity*. By this she means that proponents of demography and vital statistics in the nineteenth century attempted to insert themselves discursively into the context of governmental and scientific requirements by challenging existing academic and administrative orders

---

5 Incidentally, Gieryn calls the demarcation of science from other cultural phenomena (what he defines as "boundary work") "cultural cartography" (Gieryn 1999: 12 *passim*). The idea to combine the integrating and demarcating aspects of semantics of science comes from Kaldewey (2013: 105ff.).

and by negotiating "new disciplinary categories and projects" (Schweber 2006: 2). To pursue her vague and shifting object, she draws on what she calls "minimal definitions" of both disciplines, which include "the historic use of terms and labels to delineate a type of [...] knowledge activity" and "the professional trajectories of key figures identified with those labels" (Schweber 2006: 9). This allows her to trace the developments of demography and vital statistics as the competition between different styles of doing science in the broader institutional contexts that determined the place and role of the disciplines. My own historical sociology, instead of adhering to the conventional periodization of medical historiography, tries to follow those actors and the "professional trajectories" that have significantly reformed the understanding of science's role for medicine. These include those trajectories established by institutional actors like the NIH and other agencies. As Schweber notes, such an approach seems akin to Bruno Latour's (1987) call to "follow the scientists" to explore the assemblage of elements involved in creating scientific "facts". But like her work, my own investigation diverges from Latour's program insofar as it follows these actors "to explore the institutional contexts in which scientists promoted their projects and sought recognition" (Schweber 2006: 10).

In my case, however, the changing names of academic medicine represent more than professional trajectories of medical science. Categories like "scientific medicine" and "biomedicine" also constitute key concepts in academic and science policy discourses (Kaldewey/Schauz 2018). While Schweber is mostly interested in how the scientific styles and topics of demography and vital statistic reflected given social and political contexts, it would be too narrow to understand the academic discipline of medicine only as the result of the rhetorical and ideological positioning of medical science in a cultural space vis-à-vis social and political demands. As basic concepts in public discourses, these medical categories necessarily also constitute seemingly "objective" descriptions through which people in our society understand and communicate about science and medicine. In other words, not only have they been shaped by historical circumstance, but they also condition our expectations of academic medicine because of the co-production of science and social order (Jasanoff 2004). In other words, terms like "scientific medicine" or "biomedicine" have attached to them promises – or at least ideas – of what science and medicine, both together and individually, can do. One aim of this book, therefore, is to grant insights into a tacit dimension of our current, vibrant discourse on biomedicine and the relationship between medicine and science more generally, especially given the overgrown expectations and corresponding disappointments in current academic and science policy debates over stem cells, genomics and other high-tech applications of research to medical problems.

Works in a relatively recent interdisciplinary field of social and historical research, which studies the conceptual language of science, technology and innovation, have shown how key terms in academic and science policy discourses like "pure science", "technology" or "basic and applied research" were in fact hotly contested and the product of historical contingency (e.g., Godin 2017, Kaldewey 2013, Phillips 2012, Schatzberg 2018, Schauz 2020). As identity-markers for specific professional self-images, it is apt to assume that concepts like "scientific medicine" or "biomedicine" were constructed in discussions over the social attributes and expectations of medical science and endowed with special values and motives. The sociologist David Kaldewey (2013) coined the notion of "identity work" to describe these discursive practices: in order to sustain their scientific pursuits, researchers over the centuries balanced their professional autonomy with the expectations and values of stakeholders in society. Applied to the notion of disciplinary identity, this means that I will need to examine the professional trajectories behind basic concepts like "scientific medicine" for their integration of institutional and epistemic autonomy with simultaneous displays of practical and societal usefulness. Consequently, "scientific medicine" and "biomedicine" not only embody given institutional contexts, but they have also since conditioned how and what to expect of science and medicine.

In her study of demography and vital statistics, Schweber's main motivation is to disassociate the idea of discipline formation from its more traditional sociological conception as university-centered and intellectually autonomous. She instead places the histories of demography and vital statistics into the context of state policy and administration, showing that disciplinary activity was mainly driven by problem-oriented questions and the need to develop statistics as a tool to be applied for public health or population governance (Schweber 2006: 128ff.). This is quite novel, given the often-biased understanding of disciplines in the literature that associates them with self-centered "silos", ignorant of any practical problems or applied concerns (Jacobs 2013). My own investigation, though, seeks to place medical science – and its disciplinary activities – into the *academic* context of Germany and the USA. I share Schweber's emphasis on disciplines as also shaped by practical concerns. But I am interested in asking how conflicting notions of medical science as a place of "pure" inquiry conditioned the formation of the academic discipline, next to concerns with "applied" problems. Authors have dubbed this "a symmetrical approach that avoids any bias towards specific notions and valuations of either side of the [pure/applied] distinction" (Schauz/Kaldewey 2018: 7). The idea of an autonomous and self-centered discipline, in other words, is not more ideological than the notion of a discipline oriented to practical problems. Accordingly, I ask: what symbolic acts, basic concepts and discursive practices did protagonists employ in order to integrate the understanding of an autonomous scientific discipline with the orientation of medical science towards practical problems of clinical medicine? How did this tension between an intellectually "pure" science and societal expectations of usefulness reflect in the representations of research practices and epistemologies in medical science as well as the self-understanding of medical scientists? How has this influenced the organization of medical science as an academic institution?

By observing the disciplinary identity work (Roth 2022) of medical science, I will show how actors grappled with the issue of linking their discipline to the needs of medical practice in various ways. The tensions that developed between their ideals of an autonomous academic science and the visions for a science serving society's requirement for health care, has in popular discourses dominantly – so I argue – shaped the identity of modern academic medicine.[6] The culmination of these efforts, as Butler rightly suggests in his *Nature* article, is our modern discipline of biomedical science, although its origins lie further back than the emergence of molecular biology in the mid-20th century. I want to show how, over time, the actions of disciplinary identity-making produced semantic layers that still inform our understanding of science and medicine today. The name "biomedicine", as already indicated, transports the sense of a necessary connection between the production of biological knowledge and the application of that knowledge in clinical settings. Biomedicine has developed the ability to include in its meaning a range of different – and conflicting – scientific engagements in clinics, laboratories, hospitals and research institutions across the world. The aim of my historical sociology of medicine as a scientific discipline is to give a genealogy of this ability;

---

6 This approach is not meant to deny the significance of the medical practitioner's perspective. It is undoubted that for the patient this constitutes the crucial view. But it is meant to suggest that if we want to understand the general idea of academic medicine, we need to apply a sociological perspective to the institutions of *scientific* practice in medicine, rather than to those for the actions of medical practitioners.

to expound what I call biomedicine's *linear legacy*, and to explain why the idea of biomedicine appears to need repairing in the present discourses.

II. The Forgotten Disciplinary Identity of Medicine

Why has the sociological and historical literature up until now mostly turned a blind eye on medicine as a modern academic discipline? Answering this question has to do with how authors have portrayed the institutional relationship between the culture of medical science and the clinical profession in the transition from a medieval and early modern to a modern society. Their portrayals all revolve around constructing a more or less sharp distinction between the professional interests of science and medicine (Sturdy 2011). As historian Thomas Broman persuasively argues in his book *The Transformation of German Academic Medicine*, around 1800, "the medical profession became in effect two different occupations, one pursuing research in academic institutions, the other filling roles as district and town medical officers and bedside healers" (1996: 161, see also Broman 1989). But as our discussion of translational research indicates, their relationship is far more ambivalent. Nevertheless, a general tendency in the literature is to use this separation as an indicator for the reduction of medicine's identity to that of a modern profession, while outsourcing the history of medical science to that of the biosciences. Here, I want to briefly highlight representative works from the sociological and historical literature to demonstrate how their explanations of the differentiation of science and medical practice largely obscures the disciplinary identity of medicine.

From the Middle Ages until early Modernity medicine was one of the three higher faculties together with law and theology. The pre-modern or early modern university was one oriented mostly towards vocational education in the disciplines of the higher faculties, while the scientific subjects of the faculty of philosophy were offered as propaedeutics (Stichweh 1994: 281).[7] During this time, physicians – just like jurists and theologians

---

7 It should be noted that, although directed at vocational training, education in the three higher faculties was nevertheless highly academic. The aim for medicine was to make students proficient in the ways of academic discourse on medical topics, not in clinical practice. As Broman notes: "the centerpiece of medical education [in the eighteenth century] remained the spoken and written word" (Broman 1996: 30).

– were both researchers and practitioners, who contributed to academic discourses and treated patients (French 2003).[8] In contrast to the large share of practitioners of craft medicine, who did not enjoy a university education, these actors belonged to the small elite of learned professions that remained closely tied to the university, particularly as readers and professors of academic medicine (Broman 1996: 26ff.). As I will explain in more detail later in chapter 3, during this time, physicians regarded themselves foremost as scholars devoted to academic subjects, and only secondarily as practitioners. Stated differently, a major part of their professional identity was determined by academic rather than clinical credentials.

The structural relationship between university, science and professions changed dramatically with the turn from the eighteenth to the nineteenth century. In the process, the university became a place of research and teaching (as opposed to vocational training in law, medicine and theology as well as philosophy and mathematics) and externalized the system of professions (Stichweh 1984, 1994). Sociologist Rudolf Stichweh (1994) examined how these processes of differentiation determined a new relationship between the professions and the emerging academic disciplines. He states that with the turn of the nineteenth century the relationship between the higher faculties and the lower faculty of philosophy was exactly reversed, "by facilitating the formation of a comprehensive system of scientific disciplines and subordinating the professional knowledge systems [of law, medicine and theology] as cases of applying scientific knowledge and of developing practice-oriented bodies of knowledge" (ibid: 282).[9] At this point, the philosophical faculty and its subject areas of natural history and natural philosophy began to differentiate into modern disciplines like physics, chemistry or biology (Cahan 2003). While these became the occupation of full-time scholars, the three original professions started orienting themselves towards an interaction with clients. This resulted in the

---

8 Before the nineteenth century, patient care was vastly different from what people are accustomed to today. As part of the learned profession, physicians treated only a small circle of patients of the upper class or nobility. Doctors did not primarily treat acute ailments. They were counsellors in a wide range of physical, dietary and even ethical matters. They maintained close relationships with their elite patients and offered council mainly through the post: "The letters between doctor and his patients exchanged civilities, inquiries after health and doings of friends and family members, notifications of gifts about to be sent and of gifts gratefully received" (Shapin 2012: 308).

9 All translations from the German are my own, unless otherwise indicated.

"professional faculties, even under German conditions, approximating the character of special schools", according to Stichweh (1994: 282).

Stichweh offers a compelling argument for the close structural relationship between disciplines and professions in the context of the modern research university (something that he bemoaned as lacking in the sociological literature; Stichweh 1994: 278ff). Nevertheless, from his ideas it is difficult to locate what has become of the academic identity of medical actors in the modern university. He explains how special subjects of medicine, like pathology, have constituted themselves as scientific disciplines and how we must furthermore recognize the differentiation of special subjects into clinical and scientific research disciplines (ibid: 312). But with the general distinction between practice-oriented and "pure" bodies of knowledge he reiterates the biased understanding of disciplines as places for only those forms of scientific inquiry that operate freely and without any orientation towards clients. "Disciplines are relatively self-sufficient social systems, which are primarily concerned with internal operations and otherwise [spend time] observing their internal scientific environment" (ibid: 310). From this it would follow that all non-practically oriented research work, even if conducted in medical schools and faculties of medicine, is performed by scientists with non-medical identities. But is it reasonable to assume that all research conducted without practical aims in medical faculties is done by "outside" researchers who do not identify with medicine? Must we not also grant medical researchers the possibility of assuming "purely" scientific identities? Or, conversely, that researchers on basic mechanisms can also adopt a medical identity?

A different but complementary line of argument can be found in the historical literature. Here, authors see that with the development of the modern university former medical subjects of a "pure" sort now began assuming a biological identity and consequently belonged to the biology departments of the philosophical faculty. Like Stichweh, the explanations here also follow sociological ideas about the institutional separation of theoretical and practical medicine. With it, a modern division of labor between scientific and clinical work was introduced that still defines the medical enterprise today (Bynum 1994: 94f.). The explanation draws on what Broman states about medical practitioners increasingly regarding themselves as belonging to either one or the other sphere and therefore also beginning to operate according to separate principles. Next to the practicing physicians who consulted with patients in matters of illness and health, some doctors now worked only as full-time researchers and academic teachers, and no longer as practitioners of medicine (Broman

1996, see also Fye 1987). The assumption appears to be that since they no longer functioned as active healers, they consequently also shed their medical identity.

As Sturdy observes, in front of this institutional division of labor, historians over the past thirty or forty years have been examining the history of science and medicine with a great deal of scepticism towards the instrumental role of science for clinical practice (see also Warner 1985, 1995). This has had considerable consequences for medical historiography. In his review of the literature, he reflects on several themes through which historians have elaborated on the "inherent tension between the professional interests of science and medicine", identifying how scholars have mainly taken an "agonistic view of professionalisation and discipline formation" (Sturdy 2011: 743). Most of these works attest to a rather strict separation of the professional trajectories of medical science and clinical practice. "If the proper aim of scientific disciplines is independence, any activities that serve other disciplinary or professional agendas must represent a diversion from that aim" (ibid: 742).

This exclusivity furthermore reveals the rather traditional notion of disciplines underlying the argument. Authors have reflected on the introduction of the culture of laboratory science and experimental techniques into academic medicine as a means for actors to emancipate themselves from practical medicine and to consolidate their independent scientific endeavors:

> "Thus[,] early work on the culture of laboratory science sought among other things to elucidate the means by which scientists asserted their independence from medicine [...] and the creation of laboratories, equipped with sophisticated measuring instruments and other technologies of control, as sites both for the pursuit of experimental research and for the reproduction of disciplinary culture through training of new recruits" (ibid: 745).

In this line of argument, the emancipation from clinical practice is taken as the simultaneous emancipation from medicine as such. This has contributed to obscuring medicine's disciplinary identity by equating the role of non-practicing full-time researchers in medical faculties with the professional trajectories of other disciplines, especially with that of biology.

This effect of changing from a medical to a biological identity is most clearly visible in works dealing with the history of scientific ideas. In the scholarly literature on nineteenth-century science and medicine, actors who employed the laboratory and experiment as a means to distinguish themselves from the culture of medical practice are presented as the case for an emerging biological identity displacing its medical origins. The transitional period of the German university system around 1800 marks an important episode for historians and philosophers of science, when the old fields of natural history and natural philosophy turned into programs preconfiguring modern day disciplines like chemistry or biology (Cahan 2003, see also Stichweh 1984). In this context, many historians of science and medicine have told the story of physiology, the fundamental field of nineteenth century medical science – which I will be looking at in more detail in chapter 3 – almost exclusively with a view to our present-day life sciences (e.g., Broman 1996, Hagner 2003, Kremer 2009, Zammito 2018, see also Nyhart 1995). This form of presentism, too, has contributed to overshadowing the modern disciplinary identity of medicine.

In in his magnum opus *The Gestation of German Biology*, for example, historian of ideas and philosopher of science John Zammito (2018) traces the maturation of a scientific current over the course of the eighteenth and early-nineteenth century, later to form the basis of the modern life sciences. He argues that the appearance of the term "biology" "around 1800 signaled a theoretical and methodological *convergence* of natural history with medical physiology in comparative (i.e., *zoological*) physiology that resulted in the field of developmental morphology" (Zammito 2018: 2). Natural history was characterized by the method of observation and by the organization and classification of natural objects into a relational order to reveal the similarities and differences between different species and kinds (Pickstone 2000: 10f.). The umbrella term medical physiology, in turn, incorporated two meanings at the turn of the nineteenth century: as anatomy, it meant the study of the structures, and as physiology proper, of the life processes of higher organisms. As I will show later, the strictly physiological approach was traditionally distinguished by its focus on the theoretical reasoning about the (invisible) life processes on the basis of empirical observations made through the practical art of anatomy. Therefore, in the first half of the nineteenth century, physiology and anatomy were not yet clearly distinguished institutionally (Cunningham 2002, 2003).

According to Zammito, as physiology began incorporating "developmental and genetic accounts", next to its theories of structures and processes, and natural history was reaching beyond classifications "to explain and generalize its findings", both subsequently merged into the same research questions; namely, relating descent to organic formation in systematic accounts (Zammito 2018: 3). The resulting morphological approach constituted a field of zoology concerned with the scientific investigation of animal form. It differed from the classificatory method of natural history in that it transcended the mere comparison and descriptions of animals' anatomies and "engaged some of the central philosophical mysteries of biology" (Nyhart 1995: 2).

I will not go into any more detail about nineteenth-century physiological science here. It suffices to recognize that the intellectual developments which Zammito describes were indeed marked by a radical shift in disciplinary identities. And after about mid-century, they were followed by the founding of independent professorships for zoology with a morphological approach in the philosophical faculty or in existing natural science departments (Nyhart 1995: 90f.). But his view suggests that a general shift occurred through which physiology, as the fundamental science of academic medicine, completely changed its identity from a medical to a biological research culture. Animal morphologists or morphological zoologists were, in the most part, descendants of medical science, even though they began to receive chairs in the faculty of philosophy after mid-century. However, most of their early proponents did not yet occupy independent zoological chairs. "Instead, they taught physiology in a medical faculty, together with zoology and comparative anatomy" (Nyhart 1995: 98). In other words, before later generations became independent biologists, their precursors retained a medical identity – only some of them would later substitute this for a disciplinary identity in the life sciences. They did so while embracing the new methods of the laboratory sciences and experimental research. But it has remained largely unacknowledged that their heirs today also operate the field of biomedical research.

There is, then, a general bias in the literature that protagonists in the early decades of the century, while still situated under the roof of the medical faculty, had cognitively emancipated themselves from academic medical theory and retained but little (if any) interest in practical matters of medicine. In this regard, Broman speaks of the "professionalization" of "those communities of university-based researchers" in medicine, but he concludes that only the ones pursuing the morphological approach were also the ones defending science against demands for clinical utility (Broman 1996: 194, see also 186ff.). Since all other medical actors must therefore have remained practicing physicians, his conclusion, too, enforces the biased idea of an identity-shift from medicine to biology with the emergence of the modern research university – the thesis of "the decisive continuity", which ran from the founders of zoology in the late-eighteenth century through medical Romantics to the generation of early-nineteenth century physiologists, including Johannes Müller and his disciples, Matthias Schleiden and Theodor Schwann, the inventors of cell theory, "with whom no one can doubt that biology as a special science had taken form" (Zammito 2018: 340).

Did all medical actors who adhered to laboratory science really shed their medical identities after the mid-nineteenth century? Where was medical science institutionally located after the emergence of modern zoology and morphology? Historian Lynn Nyhart calls our attention to the fact that, before the first chairs of morphological zoology were established after mid-century, we are dealing almost exclusively with medical protagonists. Some had begun specializing in questions of animal morphology after the turn to the nineteenth century, while others later began adhering to physicalist physiology – that is, an approach strongly oriented towards vivisectional experiments and the quantitative measurement of life processes with the aid of physical and chemical techniques (Nyhart 1995: 65–102). Nonetheless, these actors retained their identities as *medical* scientists. Nyhart thus warns her readers of historians' anachronistic projection that makes these specializations *within* the discipline (of medicine) into competing factions *between* disciplines: "At the time, the difference was seen as one between two approaches within physiology; it was only in the wake of the institutional divisions following the mid-1850s that the story began to be rewritten into one between physiologists and morphologists, that is, between people inside and outside [medical] physiology" (ibid: 74). My book sets out to demonstrate how the experimental researchers with medical identities prevailed also after the 1850s and how they were able to maintain and expand a scientific discipline of medicine. Coming from physiology, this discipline did have a close biological resemblance, but actors painstakingly distinguished it as an autonomous academic endeavor from biology by tailoring it to expectations of medicine and health care. I will show how this tension between science and practice was reinterpreted in changing historical situations, how it has structured the scientific pursuit of medicine and how this is visible in our modern idea of biomedicine.

III. Historical Semantics and Discourse Analysis – Theoretical Approach and Method

I have developed my investigation into case studies organized around the basic concepts that were central for understanding medical science in Germany and the United States in particular eras – medicine as *Wissenschaft*, *wissenschaftliche Medicin*, scientific medicine, biomedicine,[10] and evidence-based medicine and translational research. The aim is to examine how these concepts were employed by actors in the historical discourses; how they were aligned programmatically in academic science and medicine; what the cultural backgrounds and interests were of protagonists that employed them; what sort of expectations they generated for the idea of medicine as a scientific discipline vis-à-vis medical practice and education, the clinic, science or society more broadly; and how the concepts were adopted in public and political discourses. I want to show how observing the use and popularization of these categories can point to moments in which some of the central cultural and social structures for academic medicine and for the system of science as we know it today were laid. Things like the requirement for physicians to receive extensive practical laboratory training; the culture of clinical science practiced today in university hospitals and clinical research centers; the rise of government interest in biomedical research; or the belief that advancing investigations into basic biological mechanisms will contribute substantially to the improvement of physical wellbeing.

In contrast to Schweber, my investigation is not strictly a *comparative* study of institutional developments – such as the development of medical specialization in international perspective (e.g., Weisz 2006). While there are of course resemblances in the developments of both countries, I have chosen a focus on Germany and the United States for specific reasons: Germany is arguably the homeland of the modern research university, which emerged at the turn of the nineteenth century (McClelland 1980, Stichweh 1984). It is from here that the idea of medicine as a scientific discipline, as it reflects in contemporary biomedical research, originates. Accordingly, the development of medical science needs to be situated in this context. However, it is from United States policy discourses that the idea of biomedicine emanated, which requires also looking at the social history of the academic system in the United States. According to Stichweh, American Universities went through a similar development as the German ones, only a century later (Stichweh 1994: 282f.). As we will see, US actors took inspiration from the German role model, but created their own idea of academic research institutions. This therefore also requires looking at how the scientific discipline of medicine developed differently in this cultural context at the start of the twentieth century, and how

---

10 I am keeping with the conventional term here, although the historical phrase – as I will demonstrate in chapter 6 – was "biomedical science".

it prepared the invention of biomedicine – a category that has become universal today. Beginning in Germany during the Romantic Era, I will first examine the creation of a modern disciplinary identity of academic medicine, which becomes refined around mid-century. European academic ideals are subsequently exported to the United States, where a vastly different American version of scientific medicine forms during the Progressive Era, which then ultimately lays the ground for the discipline of biomedical science in the post-war discourse.[11]

Methodologically, my study draws on historical semantics (or conceptual history) and discourse analysis. Discourse analysis is the apt approach to deal with such a vast and complex topic because it affords studying the issue of discipline formation from a relatively comfortable distance and without the burden of detailed comprehensiveness. Instead, the specific historical cases, which I examine, are representative of the regularities that governed how social phenomena were perceived and understood at a given time as well as of the hidden strategies that applied to making culturally comprehensible statements. They can therefore reveal the semantic complexity underneath the conceptual condensations, which constitute a society's systems of thought and communication about science and medicine.

One such structuring regularity in scientific discourse, for instance, is "credibility", as Gieryn (1995, 1999) shows. What constitutes credibility is historically contingent, but in what he calls "boundary work", scientific actors resort to different discursive strategies to manifest their authority over making truth claims regarding a given phenomenon. "Epistemic authority does not exist as an omnipresent ether, but rather is enacted as people debate (and ultimately decide) where to locate the legitimate jurisdiction over natural facts" (Gieryn 1999: 15). Boundary work gets employed for pursuing professional goals and interests; it is used to demarcate science from religion, technology or "pseudoscience" as well as for distinguishing scientific disciplines, which becomes manifest in antonyms such as "pure" and "applied science" (Schauz 2020: 47, see also Kaldewey 2013: 322ff.). In my book, the dominant form of boundary work is that of assigning credibility to scientific statements and practices concerning clinical facts.

---

11 While I employ a wide temporal scope (from the turn of the eighteenth to the nineteenth century until the present), my study accordingly only highlights important episodes in which the basic understanding of medicine as a scientific discipline was refined in the context of changing institutional or social developments.

Boundary work is a widely used approach in science and technology studies (STS) that can also help explain conflicts over policy influence (e.g., Greenhalgh 2008). As historian Désirée Schauz notes, boundary work discourses help seeing that such demarcations are contested and always up for grabs by the actors involved (Schauz 2020: 47). She also notes how Gieryn, even though his studies include historical cases, is hardly interested "in long-term semantic changes and the specific historical manifestations of demarcation concepts" (ibid.). To meet this interest, therefore, it requires a conceptual history approach, which is compatible with the idea of discourses on boundary work (see also Kaldewey 2013). Conceptual history is a scholarly tradition most closely associated with the historian Reinhart Koselleck (1979, 2006), who in a combination of intellectual and social history investigated how changes in language also reflect historical changes. His aim was to show how key concepts in the modern political and social language of Europe became consolidated between about 1750 and 1850 as expressions of specific experiences in relation to social expectations. The conceptual approach has subsequently been expanded to a variety of different intellectual fields (see Müller/Schmieder 2016, Wimmer 2015).

In the social studies of science, technology and innovation, the methodology has been used to productively show that "concepts such as basic and applied research are heatedly contested, while at the same time remain[ing] indispensable and of persistent relevance for communicating science policy" (Schauz/Kaldewey 2018: 7). With this approach, concepts can be understood as simultaneously embodying "cognitive strategies designed to deal with reality", and as expressions of human experience like "expectations pointing to desirable or, alternatively, dreaded futures" (ibid: 10). I will show how actors connected to medical science employed their concepts not as neutral categories but rather to define experiences in academic medicine from the background of their values and interests. Fundamental concepts can be seen to have started as subjective categories, used as rallying cries to defend a cause or publicly legitimize the maintenance of a cultural identity. Only upon successful implementation as an accepted category can they be regarded as having received analytical value as an expression of reality. Thus, instead of treating modern concepts as categories, which somehow objectively periodize the history of medicine, I am here instead interested in the question of actors' perceptions and conceptualizations of the relationship between science, medicine and society more generally. In a very basic sense, therefore, I want to assume that protagonists deployed new basic concepts to try and force society to comprehend the reality of science and medicine in their terms.

Key concepts in the academic discourses are also crucial for ordering society's understanding and expectations of medical science. On the one hand, as I have noted already, they work to integrate often irreconcilable activities in different disciplines or institutions into Harris' (2005) notion of a supercategory. As science studies scholars employing the conceptual approach have aptly demonstrated, key concepts like "natural science", "pure science", or "basic" and "applied research", provide unifying narratives that work to reconcile into a coherent picture the seeming opposition between the meanings of science as an autonomous *and* as a socially relevant pursuit (Bud 2014, Clarke 2010, Kaldewey 2013: 311–410, Kaldewey/Schauz 2018, Phillips 2012, Schauz 2020). Narratives, such as the one stating that disinterested basic research will at some unspecified time in the future lead to useful outcomes, then incorporate both the self-understanding of academic science as well as attributions stemming from societal expectations.

For me, consequently, this means investigating the key medical categories for the narratives they provide, which paint into a coherent picture the conflicting ideas of what it means to pursue medicine as an autonomous academic science and as a contribution to health care.[12] Since these categories incorporate both the notion of an autonomous academic pursuit and of medical usefulness, they also linguistically integrate both our understanding of medicine as a profession and as a scientific discipline.[13]

More, basic concepts are highly relevant for the organization and categorization of scientific practices and fields. Thus, situated in the discourse opposed to other categories, they are also connected to a dimension of what science studies scholar Steven Shapin calls "metascientific statements": overarching expressions made about the nature and purpose of science, which are generally not defenses of science as a uniform and global operation, but rather "local criticisms of certain tendencies *within* science, or within parts of it – criticisms that are often substantial and

---

12 I will not be able to consider here how *materiality* plays a crucial role in conditioning these narratives, but only on the narratives themselves. Nonetheless, I find the issue of materiality to be an important question to pursue in future research.

13 Thus, from this integrative perspective, one can understand why our cultural idea of medicine is less shaped by the actions and experiences of medical practitioners than it is by the provisions for medical practice provided by scientific knowledge.

vehemently expressed" (2012: 44, see also Kaldewey 2013: 107, Schauz 2020: 21). The organization and classification of the work conducted under the supercategorical umbrella using scientific or medical categories always also implies situating these activities within a normative hierarchy. Fundamental concepts in the academic and science policy discourses thus ultimately give an indication of "the permanent negotiations over different interests, epistemic and social goals and norms, institutional and financial arrangements and their related expectations and experiences of science" (Schauz 2015: 57). How actors employed key concepts as at the same time discursively reconciling and conflicting linguistic elements accordingly helps observe the distinctions and fault lines, which ran through the academic system at a given moment.

craft medicine	medical practice		medical theory
——————————————————— *early modern understanding* ———————————————————			
medico-surgery	Kunst (art)		Wissenschaften (sciences)
——————————————————————— *Romantic Era* ———————————————————————			
	Internal medicine & surgery		*Wissenschaft*
applied science			**pure science**
——————————————————— *mid-nineteenth century Germany* ———————————————————			
clinical medicine	scientific medicine	rational medicine	physiological medicine
——————————————————— *Progressive Era (United States)* ———————————————————			
clinical science			preclinical sciences
——————————————————————— *twenty-first century discourse* ———————————————————————			
medical practice	**applied science**		**basic science**
evidence-based medicine	translational science		biomedicine

Table 1.3: Semantic field of modern medicine in Germany and the USA in the context of changing ideologies of science (my depiction).

The concepts in the historical discourses of medicine that form the subject of my investigation are related to each other synchronically and diachronically in a wider semantic field (Kaldewey 2013: 176–185, see also figure 1.3). The theory of semantic fields holds that meaning is not reducible to single words but that it constitutes itself in the way that concepts relate to each other in similarity, in opposition, or in hierarchies of sense. Therefore, my book not only examines the key concepts that characterize the discourses themselves, but also looks at important categories that relate to these, such as other basic concepts like "pure science" or "basic research", various notions of scientific and clinical method, medical (sub-)disciplines like physiology or pathology, the scientific discipline of biology, the clinic and others.

To grasp the relations between these meanings and terms, however, it requires to differentiate linguistically between a level of expression and a level of content. For this purpose, conceptual history employs an *onomasiological* perspective on the one side and *semasiological* one on the other (Koselleck 1979: 121). The rationale behind this distinction is that only looking at changes in linguistic meanings of single terms over time would constitute an insufficient analysis of the history of fundamental concepts. Rather, I also consider how *different* designations at various times meant the same thing factually. This is somewhat akin to Schweber's minimal definitions of vital statistics and demography. "The onomasological approach assumes that there is a given phenomenon or idea that has been described with different terms in the course of history in different contexts" (Kaldewey 2018: 163f.). From this angle, it becomes apparent how, in a diachronic perspective, ideas have prefigured or resembled the concepts, which have only subsequently become coined as the terms of interest for my analysis. For instance, the changing description of medicine from the Latin *scientia* to the German *Wissenschaft* reveals the "general cultural shift" (ibid.), which substituted the idea of medicine as a premodern body of philosophical knowledge with the idea of medicine as a modern scientific institution.

The semasiological approach, in contrast, enables an examination of "what a given term denotes in different contexts and how its meaning changes over time" (ibid.). It lets me perceive how actors employed the same term to express different things in different periods; for example, that the term "medicine" could mean a practical art for medieval and a scientific discipline for modern actors, while it is understood mostly as a professional practice in the present. In relation, the translation of a term also alters its meaning across the concerned language boundaries. Historian Denise Phillips (2015) alludes to how the rendering of the German "Wissenschaft" into the English word "science" in the second half of the nineteenth century changed the meaning of the word significantly due to the cultural and political differences between actors in Germany and Great Britain.[14] The sense of the word "wissenschaftliche Medicin" or "scientific medicine" varied considerably with the change from the German to the American cultural context, as I will show in chapters 4 and 5. In sum, a look at the semantic field surrounding key concepts allows for studying the changing disciplinary identity of medicine through the changing designations, meanings and tropes with which the idea of medicine as a science was inscribed into the scientific system. The analysis is about discourses on how different institutions of medical science and neighboring fields were related or conflicted with each other, how they were organized in the academic system and how they were legitimized in front of society.

Empirically, my research draws on a mix of primary and secondary sources. It concerns the discursive identity work of actors in and around academic medicine in Germany and the USA. I accordingly investigate historical sources that offer programmatic statements about the role and purpose of science for medicine and health care and that have popularized the use of key concepts, such as "scientific medicine", "clinical science" or "biomedical science". My investigation concentrates on documents that contain depictions by actors involved in the construction of academic medicine's self-understanding and public image. In analogy to Schauz' pursuit of the meaning of the natural sciences over the centuries, I want to regard that "[a]ll discourses are principally relevant in which expectations on science [and medicine] are expressed, be it that societal actors addressed them to scientists [directly] or that researchers have communicated them with a view to their own work" (Schauz 2020: 43). For this purpose, I have selected those sources in which the historical discourse can be said to have become condensed. My investigation draws on documents that were at the center of crucial semantic transitions – important and influential historical texts in specialized journals, innovative speeches and memoranda or policy papers about standpoints in medicine with respect to science.

My study is then also aided by the available historiographical literature that has reconstructed the state of German and US science and medicine. I have consulted texts that examine them especially in the academic context of the two countries. Naturally, it would be quite impossible for me to work through all the relevant historical data spanning two centuries and

---

14 The most striking difference is that "Wissenschaft" has a far more encompassing meaning, which includes humanities next to the natural sciences, whereas "science" is restricted to natural science fields.

two countries that a myriad of historical studies has brilliantly processed. For this reason, I have not only restricted myself to specific time periods to design the individual cases of my study, but also mainly analyzed "newer" historiographical literature on medicine in Germany and the USA for their contribution to a conceptual and institutional history of medical science as a discipline. Especially the works that have developed since the 1970s and 1980s, when the history of medicine increasingly became a domain of professional historians, has proven as relevant to my questions about the production of medicine's disciplinary identity (Löwy 2011, see also Rheinberger 2009).

However, my research design requires applying a certain measure of caution to the literature. We cannot trust at the outset that historians always reflect on the semantic heritage of the key concepts they themselves employ. Like the historical actors they study, their work is also conditioned by prevailing social values and conventions. For example, Harris shows in his book that the term "science" became widely used only in the seventeenth century, but that it is "applied retrospectively" to describe many forms of scholarly activity since at least the time of Aristotle (Harris 2005: 25). Through this practice, however, premodern concepts get endowed with modern characteristics that were still largely foreign to them, thereby also ignoring the cultural shifts that accompanied the use of new vocabularies. So, when historians employ terms like "biomedical" in the context of nineteenth-century academic medicine, it needs to be remembered that they are not referring to the postwar category. Instead, they are anachronistically projecting our present understanding of science and medicine back onto the past, distorting the meaning of the concept at hand.

The same caution also holds for the analytical categories that historians use. A salient example is the concept of "scientific medicine", which, next to biomedicine, plays a central role in my book. Historians of science and medicine in the 1970s and 1980s began composing nuanced studies about the ideological, cultural, professional, social, political and economic role of science in medicine. These were intended to revise the rather positivistic ideas of science and medicine of their predecessors (see Warner 1985). One unintended consequence of this new current in medical histo-riography was the transformation of scientific medicine from a concept used by historical actors at a given time and in a specific place into a universal category. As historian John Harley Warner stated in an extensive review-essay of the Anglo-American medical history literature, published in the 1995 volume of *Osiris*, it was perceived, at the time, that "the notion of *scientific medicine* stands among the sturdiest bastions of presentism in the field" (Warner 1995: 188, see also 1985: 50, 57). The complaint arose from the term being, to a large extent, used in the literature to describe only that from of "medicine rooted in experimental laboratory science" (ibid.). The impulse of revisionists was that the idea of medicine as being "scientific" should be applied equally to all understandings in which medical actors at different times and in different places referred to scientific practices. For Anglo-American historians the idea of scientific medicine thus comprises a broad understanding of science-based medical practices no longer concurrent with the historical concept, which indeed describes a laboratory-centered program.

Finally, next to providing a new perspective on the current biomedical discourse, my project also wants to contribute to the historical sociology of scientific disciplines. For this purpose, I will develop a new model of disciplines in the next chapter that combines elements worth preserving from two competing scholarly discourses – science and technology studies and "classical" sociology of science – and puts it to the test in the subsequent chapters. This model, I intend to show, on the one hand, can reveal the more fragmented and messier dimension of science that is truer to how it is practiced "on the ground". On the other, it helps preserve those important insights explaining structural aspects, which allow conceptualizing the growth and institutional differentiation of science as well as the intimate – and sometimes obscured – relation between academic education and specialized research. A view of disciplinary structures shaped as the result of discursive activities borne by professional interests in specific historical contexts, so I hope, may also provide an example for other cases to shed some new light on sciences with a long historical tradition, or also help explain how in more recent experiences the practices of actors form institutional structures.

2. For a Sociology of Disciplinary Cultures

Referring to a notion of scientific or academic disciplines[15] to describe the institutions of science has today become somewhat marginal in science studies discourses, particularly in science and technology studies (STS). Originally, the concept of disciplines was used in an institutional approach in the sociology of science, which linked the formal organization of a scientific community to a set of shared norms and rules for scientific practice (see Roth 2022). In this context, disciplines were regarded as providing vital social infrastructures for the coordination of scientific knowledge production on different levels.

Instead of answering questions about the formal organization of *science*, however, STS has a long tradition of focusing on the messy constitution of *research* practices (Felt et al. 2017: 8ff., 21ff.). Already in the 1970s, with the influence of the Sociology of Scientific Knowledge (SSK), which introduced the principle of studying scientific failure and success symmetrically by looking at social factors, science studies scholars turned away from investigating formal structures toward the social and discursive practices of science, thereby sidelining investigations of disciplinary formation (e.g., Barnes et al. 1996, see also Schweber 2006: 15). Beginning with the 1980s, through pioneering ethnographical work in research laboratories, STS revealed the scientific enterprise to be a messy and heterogeneous business not easily compartmentalized into homogenous scientific disciplines (e.g., Latour/Woolgar 1986, Knorr Cetina 1981). Though practices in research cultures also follow rules, these do not primarily derive from scientific epistemologies or "paradigms" (Kuhn 2012) as the institutional tradition claimed. Instead, they are seen as determined by the local sociotechnical conditions of research laboratories.[16]

Next to a concentration on research cultures instead of scientific disciplines, some authors in the field furthermore contend that the system

---

15 I will be using the terms "scientific disciplines" and "academic disciplines" interchangeably throughout the text.

16 The Käte Hamburger Kolleg: Cultures of Research (c:o/re) at RWTH Aachen University currently provides fresh approaches to studying research cultures, charting their complex transformations in light of the digitalization of science and of pressing societal issues, such as climate change, from a philosophical, sociological and historical perspective: https://khk.rwth-aachen.de.

of science had undergone crucial structural changes in the late twentieth century. The diagnoses of the arrival of "post-normal science" (Funtowicz/Ravetz 1993) or of the switch of the scientific system to a "mode 2" of knowledge production (Gibbons et al. 1994) have contributed to an idea of disciplines as remnants of an antiquated form of science.[17] In this process, science is thought to have lost its disciplinary foundation in favor of new configurations such as inter-, multi- and transdisciplinarity – changes that seem to have been announcing themselves since the early twentieth century, when public and private institutions began housing scientific research next to the university (Ash 2019). As a result, the academic communities defining disciplines are regarded as having "become diffuse, and consequently, the university structures of faculties and departments, institutes and centres that create and sustain these communities become less relevant" (Nowotny et al. 2001: 89). If disciplines no longer play a major role in the social study of science, why then employ such a seemingly antiquated analytical concept? What distinguishes the idea of research cultures from disciplines? And why does it require that we revive the disciplinary frame to study the development of medical science?

On closer inspection, the notion of disciplines seems far from being an obsolete analytical category. Instead, scholarly discourses on the social studies of science continue to depend on the idea of scientific disciplines, although the concept has been criticized by authors for depicting a conservative image of scientific organization. While STS scholarship thus largely gives off the impression that disciplinarity, as an antiquated mode of science, can be analytically discarded, the field nevertheless continues to rely heavily on the term. In the fourth and current edition of the *Handbook of Science and Technology Studies*, a collection of contributions by leading scholars in the STS field, for example, there is indeed a chapter on the "social and epistemic organization of scientific work", although it tells readers that "studies of disciplines and specialties are written in a highly variable vocabulary" that ranges from "paradigms, social worlds, epistemic cultures" to "thought styles and cultures, ways of knowing, styles of scientific reasoning, and many more" (Hackett et al. 2017: 739). The book includes no other systematic elaboration of disciplines, nor does it

---

17 These diagnoses have subsequently been criticized for their schematic understanding of historical developments in science and for primarily deriving from political motivations rather than from genuine scientific insights (Pestre 2003, Shinn 1999, see also Kaldewey 2013: 91–101).

index the item at the end (Felt et al. 2017).[18] Somewhat surprisingly, however, given the limited space devoted to disciplines conceptually, a simple full-text search of the digital version of the *Handbook* retrieves roughly one-hundred and sixty hits for "discipline" and "disciplines".[19] Despite the availability of alternative concepts, therefore, in terms of pure figures, each of the handbook's thirty-six chapters on average references the term more than four times. It would be worth investigating whether the term is indeed always referenced negatively, in contradistinction to the inter-, multi- and transdisciplinary alternatives.

A search on the *Web of Science* for mentions in scholarly publications in the field of STS reveals a similar picture. It shows a slight but steady uptake in relative numbers for the topic of "academic" or "scientific disciplines" in leading STS journals: from about 1 % of publications referencing the concept in the early 1990s to about 5 % in the late 2010s.[20] Not only do these figures stand in stark contrast to the general theme running through much of STS, of disciplines as a largely negligible analytical category; its continued use – even increase – furthermore points to a fundamental sociological problem in the social study of science, namely, that STS lack a viable explanation of the concept of scientific or academic disciplines that transcends its use as an antithesis to multi-, inter- and transdisciplinarity.

My purpose in this chapter is to fill this lacuna by proposing a concept of disciplinary cultures that satisfies both the intellectual interests of STS and of sociological studies that focus on the formal organization of science. The crucial problem with both perspectives is that they trivialize the focus of the other tradition. Put differently, while STS emphasize the relevance and complexity of research practices, they at the same time downplay the importance of institutional structures, which ultimately enable and sustain such practices (e.g., Knorr Cetina 1999). Conversely,

---

18 The index does, however, list "interdisciplinary integration", "multidisciplinarity", and "transdisciplinary research", while an entry for "disciplines" or its equivalent is missing (Felt et al. 2017: 1169, 1173, 1188).

19 I used the extended search function in my pdf-reader to scan the digital version of the *Handbook*, searching for exact matches of the above-mentioned keywords ("scientific" and "academic discipline/s"). Results include a minimum number of mentions listed in the references of the chapters.

20 The search was conducted on February 22, 2021, and included publications in the journals *Configurations*; *Minerva*; *Science and Technology Studies*; *Science as Culture*; *Science, Technology, & Human Values*; and *Social Studies of Science* between 1991 and 2020 (n=4,624). Searches were in publication titles and abstracts and the search string was designed to eliminate hits on the topics of inter-, multi-, or transdisciplinarity as well as discipline as a concept of power formation.

while sociological studies underscore the importance of formal structures, they understate the significance of research praxis for the development of scientific institutions (e.g., Turner 2000). STS largely disregard the role of institutions for providing the necessary socialization and training of scientific recruits.[21] In turn, crucial features, such as academic education and recruitment, are largely thought of without recourse to the work going on in research facilities in sociological studies on disciplines.

The notion of disciplinary cultures, which I employ here, can function as an amendment to these complementary blind spots by providing a perspective on the interaction between local research institutions and the organizing social structures. It offers a link between concrete practices of knowledge production and global narratives of science. Such narratives not only transport societal expectations and visions of science in society, but they also have an ordering function that reflects in the formal organization of the scientific system. Think of the division of labor implied in narratives of "basic research", for example, where uninterested investigations form the platform for future applied research and implementation (Schauz 2014). Such divisions become institutionalized in faculties and university departments, determining the order of disciplines and the distribution of their jurisdictions. The narratives implied in the concept of "pure science" played an important role in ordering medical science in the nineteenth and early-twentieth century, for instance. Pure science tells the story that even epistemic objects of practical concern like clinical care need to be studied without any interest in application. This meant that medical science, even on practical matters, was kept strictly separated institutionally from the actual practice of clinical medicine. The point is that this perspective on disciplinary cultures emphasizes how both formal structure and research praxis are connected in social and cultural imaginaries of science in society (see also Jasanoff/Kim 2015). Biomedical or clinical science as disciplinary cultures, in other words, were not only designations for local programs of research praxis revolving around matters of health and disease. They also embody visions of the concrete role that medical science plays for improving clinical practice and health care more generally.

Moreover, referring to a concept that combines the notion of research cultures with the more formal understanding of disciplines overcomes one-sided concentrations on either *research* or *science*. By showing that both

---

21 By reducing the idea of science to research work, some scholars in STS do not see the university course as a crucial moment of academic socialization, acknowledging the process only as part of a mature scientific career (e.g., Felt et al. 2013).

are intimately connected via societal expectations and global narratives, there no longer is a need to distinguish analytically between the *practices* of scientists on the one side and the formal *organizations* in which they operate on the other side. Rather, such an understanding of disciplinary cultures is conceptually prolific because it shows how professional behaviors, conventions and values not only refer to research praxis, but always also convey social values, norms and convictions. Tracing the disciplinary identity work that corresponds to these cultures reveals how the representation and positioning of scientific practices always incorporates a, what today is called "research policy", dimension. Next to the rules and norms of a research culture, this also points to the institutional space of a given discipline (Roth 2022). Stated in very general terms, the decision to employ a certain method, technique or concept for knowledge production in a certain field always also entails a political decision about how to position a discipline vis-à-vis society and its expectations.

In what follows, I will be reviewing central works in the sociology of science and in STS that study the organization of science and research. I want to thereby operationalize my theoretical approach and method for the cases that follow, by highlighting the analytical concepts that inform the empirical investigation of my book. The study of the discipline of medical science, therefore, neither takes on the form of an ethnographic investigation of concrete research practices nor of a sociological theory of the formal organization of the scientific system. Instead, I will tackle the sociological-historical issue of how cultures of science create their disciplinary identity, establish themselves institutionally and legitimize themselves socially through their *(self-)depictions of work in academic and science policy discourses.*

I. Academic Knowledge and the Social Structure of Science

My study holds on to the idea of disciplines but wants to update it to be able to also capture the messy constitution of research practices central to works in STS. This is not specific to the notion of disciplines, which imply (abstract) knowledge as one of their central features. In the traditional understanding of the medieval and early modern European university, "disciplina" described the context of higher learning. It consisted of a systematic body of theoretical knowledge ("doctrina"), which was not necessarily scientific in the modern sense, and specific rules of learning that students needed to master (Stichweh 1992). Only since the turn from the eighteenth to the nineteenth century have disciplines also become places of academic research and therefore a central structural element in the modern system of science (Stichweh 1984). As a sociological concept, the institutional understanding of scientific disciplines has the important function of answering questions about how academic areas of knowledge and social structures in science are related. In what can be called "the sociology of scientific disciplines",[22] disciplines transcend the simple idea of being bodies of theoretical knowledge. Instead, in modern disciplines, specific aspects of that knowledge are connected to social functions like knowledge production or transmission. In this view, the organization of science into disciplines is largely congruent with that of university institutes and departments, where scientists advance disciplinary knowledge and secure recruitment into their ranks through formal training and by providing official credentials (Turner 2000).

Thomas S. Kuhn's (2012 [1962]) famous book *The Structure of Scientific Revolutions* proved highly influential in relating knowledge to social organization. Though it is primarily a philosophical work, it was nevertheless foundational for both STS and the sociology and history of science.[23] His notion of a paradigm, with its sociological connotation, allows to conceptualize academic disciplines as *scientific communities*. According to Kuhn, a paradigm is a central point of reference for such a community, since it provides samples or models of professional action based on past achievements (Kuhn 2012: 10ff., 175ff., see also Hacking 2012: xviiff.). Paradigms distinguish a community, because they are imperative, telling members what can be known, what issues to pursue, how to pursue them, and what can serve as legitimate methods and answers. For Kuhn, a consistently shared paradigm is the precondition for science to proceed in its everyday operations. In this mode of "normal science", scientific practice comprises mostly puzzle- and problem-solving in the still unknown areas staked out by the paradigm (Kuhn 2012: 35ff.).

His central thesis, however, is that true progress in science does not result from the aggregation of knowledge produced by the problem-solv-

---

22 The label "the sociology of scientific disciplines", adopted from a text by Rudolf Stichweh (1992) on the historical formation of disciplinary structures in the transition to the modern system of science, is, strictly speaking, *not* the name of a scholarly tradition. Rather, I use it here to group sociological works, which have made disciplines their central object of analysis (e.g., Abbott 2001, Jacobs 2013, Turner 2000, Weingart 2000).

23 See, e.g., the special section on Kuhn's influence after fifty years in *Social Studies of Science* volume 42, no. 3 (June 2012).

ing actions. Instead, it depends on the occurrence of "revolutions", in which a scientific community is placed on a completely new basis. A given paradigm only legitimizes researchers' everyday practices until they begin to encounter anomalies in their work processes – aspects not explainable within the frame of practices and norms set up by a paradigm. The more of these anomalies aggregate, the more practitioners are compelled to design and use new theories and methods that question the governing paradigm. Work according to the old paradigm becomes increasingly incommensurable with the new intellectual practices. Eventually, once the old is replaced by the new, the constitution of the academic field is fundamentally transformed: "as if the professional community had been suddenly transported to another planet where familiar objects are seen in a different light and are joined by unfamiliar ones as well." (Kuhn 2012: 111).

For the sociological understanding of disciplines, it is central that an idea of scientific communities determined by paradigms allows conceptualizing the relationship between epistemic and social structures with reference to the mechanisms of socialization and institutionalization. The social and intellectual connection between research and teaching is a fundamental principle of scientific disciplines, which will also play an important part in my study. If we conceive of disciplines as scientific communities, we can see how academic role structures are connected to the prospect of scientific careers. These bind academic recruits to a discipline and to specific research practices (Stichweh 1984: 87). Through the institutions of lectures and courses, canonical textbooks and practical training, students acquire a certain paradigm through academic socialization that guides their work. In the words of Kuhn, members of a community "have undergone similar educations and professional initiations; in the process they have absorbed the same technical literature and drawn many of the same lessons" (Kuhn 2012: 176). Accordingly, in scientific disciplines, areas of knowledge are connected to academic education and the formal organization of scientific work. They organize the academic labor market by providing formal credentials to graduates, which confirm that they possess the required means to pursue tasks in a certain academic field (Turner 2000). "A discipline is a form of social organization that generates new ideas and research findings, certifies this knowledge, and in turn teaches this subject matter to interested students" (Jacobs 2013: 28).

II. From the Culture of Science to Cultures of Research

There were major points of critique, coming especially from the STS side of science studies, against the sociological concept of disciplines. The first was that the empirical reality of research work did not confirm the neatly structured conception of science. Instead, with a view to research praxis, science appeared as a messy business. The second, as I already mentioned in the introduction, was that disciplines were seen as tending only to matters of importance to themselves, ignorant of any societal relevance and thereby barring themselves from interdisciplinary activity. I will mainly look at the first objection here since it immediately concerns the organization of science and research and the concept of disciplines. The second, in contrast, takes on the form of a normative pitting of disciplinarity against inter-, multi- and transdisciplinarity. This line of argument, though, is of little relevance for my discussion here.[24]

Kuhn had developed his theory of scientific revolutions in front of the history of physics, a very homogenous field in which there is a high degree of consensus on rules and norms. This means that his thoughts were already biased against disciplines exhibiting a range of different paradigms, rules or norms like sociology or biology. For scholars in STS, however, this older understanding of science as a monolithic and unitary institution needed to be abandoned for a new idea of science in which research, understood as a socially heterogenous and complex form of action, is the main feature of the scientific system. Thus, the study of concrete scientific practices has received special prominence in science studies, especially in order to supersede the theory- and knowledge-centered traditions of the field (Lenoir 1997: 45ff.). This induced a shift in perspective and important protagonists welcomed the departure from the investigation of the "culture of science" to examining the many "cultures of research" instead (e.g., Pickering 1992, see also Galison/Stump 1996). As Bruno Latour – a pivotal figure in STS – once programmatically explained in an article in *Science*:

> "Science is certainty; research is uncertainty. Science is supposed to be cold, straight, and detached; research is warm, involving and risky. Science puts an end to the vagaries of human disputes; research creates controversies. Science produces objectivity by escaping as much as pos-

---

24 See my brief overview of the debate in Roth (2022). Authors in the "sociology of scientific disciplines" also offer a more complementary view of disciplinarity and interdisciplinarity, rather than the oppositional view dominating STS discourses (see Abbott 2001, Jacobs 2013, Turner 2000).

sible from the shackles of ideology, passions, and emotions; research feeds on all those to render objects of inquiry familiar" (Latour 1998: 208).

The so-called laboratory studies of the 1980s helped to set the focus on research cultures instead of on science as a (homogenous) system. Through rich anthropological investigations into the work conducted in research laboratories, authors showed that "science" could be understood as something that takes place in everyday practices and in negotiations over the (mundane) technicalities of research approaches (Knorr Cetina 1981, Latour/Woolgar 1986, Lynch 1985). These studies disclosed the messy and contingent processes that preceded the orderly and unambiguous publication of scientific findings in journal papers. In fact, scientists spent most of their time manipulating their research objects or arranging their data in ways to fit the propositions they were trying to make. Most crucially for my purposes, however, this perspective on the research laboratory also revealed that the integration of scientists into communities did not happen on the basis of disciplinary affiliation or by sharing values and paradigms. Instead, it is the work on concrete problems through which researchers collectively identify themselves.

This trend was indeed revolutionary in the Kuhnian sense: it set the social and cultural research into science on a completely new footing and revealed a never-before-studied dimension of the scientific system. Despite the rejection of his theory, Kuhn's work also provided some crucial inspiration. In their iconic ethnographic study of lab work at the Salk Institute, Latour and Woolgar, for instance, see him set "the general basis for a conception of the social character of science" (Latour/Woolgar 1986: 275). Instead of focusing on the institutionalization of paradigms in the form of research chairs, lectures or textbooks, though, the authors here emphasize "the correspondence between a particular group, network, or laboratory and a complex mixture of beliefs, habits, systematized knowledge, exemplary achievements, experimental practices, oral traditions, and craft skills" (Latour/Woolgar 1986: 54). Latour and Woolgar go on to note that, although "referred to as 'culture' in anthropology, this latter set of attributes is commonly subsumed under the term paradigm when applied to people calling themselves scientists" (Latour/Woolgar 1986: 54). However, by calling it "culture" instead of "paradigm", they shift the focus from pompous scientific theories, and the rather abstract level of organizing professional behavior, to the local and quotidian activities making up research, "the set of arguments and beliefs to which there is a constant appeal in daily life and which is the object of all passions, fears, and respect" (Latour/Woolgar 1986: 55). My idea of disciplinary cultures accepts a similar mix of informal and formal, tacit and explicit knowledge forms as constitutive of groups of researchers.

Connected with this reformulation of the empirical reality of the scientific system came a further objection against the sociological concept of disciplines. This objection was directed against the general notion that disciplines were an indication of the scientific system's formal unity, since the same basic operational mechanisms were at work in every discipline (e.g., Stichweh 2007). Instead, STS and other works in science studies with a focus on practices demonstrated the disunity of science; or even that what is called science was in reality a highly fragmented patchwork of different research cultures. Karin Knorr Cetina's work on "epistemic cultures" provided a sociological foundation for this understanding of science (Knorr Cetina 1999, Knorr Cetina/Reichmann 2015).

According to Knorr Cetina, such cultures of knowledge work incorporate the complex material, social, technical and cognitive structures that guide scientific practices – the "texture" of science, which is not congruent with disciplinary differentiation and is found only in "the deep social spaces of modern institutions" (Knorr Cetina 1999: 2). This is exemplified in the idea of the laboratory, which can range from the biological workbench to the vast apparatuses of high energy physics. Knorr Cetina revealed how the ongoing messy and contingent processes making up scientific practices are regulated on a micro-social dimension particular to each individual research area (Knorr Cetina 1999: 23–45). Different from Kuhn's idea of paradigms, therefore, which described the relation between theory and professional work, the notion of "culture" receives prominence in this context because it is meant to denote more broadly "the frames of meaning within which people enact their lives"; but it is also taken on the other hand to signify the idea of a plurality of fields of research, which use "different vocabularies of knowledge" or target "different objects of study", and which also form radically unique "realties" with their own ontologies (Knorr Cetina/Reichmann 2015: 873f.). Knorr Cetina's central thesis with respect to the integration of science is therefore that, in contrast to the institutional understanding of sociology of science, the knowledge practices of contemporary science are not defined by professional or organizational interests. They are rather determined by the baselines that govern the handling of research objects and by the routines for solving technical issues that are particular to research work in a specific social and material setting.

From the idea of epistemic cultures thus emerges a picture of science that is typical also for other works with a focus on scientific praxis: in contrast to the homogenous image given by scientific disciplines, these studies emphasize the cultural fragmentation of science (Galison/Stump 1996). They emphasize the "multiplicity, patchiness, and heterogeneity of the space in which scientists work", instead of presupposing the idea "of scientific culture as a single unity" (Pickering 1992: 8). Science is portrayed as "not one enterprise but many", all of which form "a whole landscape – or market – of independent epistemic monopolies producing vastly different products" (Knorr Cetina 1999: 4).[25]

While my study supports the idea of science as being composed of a heterogenous field of different research cultures, to project them in stark isolation from one another seems exaggerated. As noted above, disciplinary cultures share an orientation to societal problems and expectations by adhering to the overarching narratives of science, i.e., even the vastly disparate fields of molecular biology and high-energy physics necessarily subscribe to popular understandings like that of basic research to justify their endeavors in front of society. As the case of medical science will show, though cultures here tended to fragment and separate from one another, they nevertheless retained an identity as *medical* research fields (sometimes even when it was hard to see their medical relevance). For me, therefore, it seems more plausible to argue for the simultaneity of the patchiness of the research culture landscape and the semantic unity of science provided by basic concepts and overarching narratives. Both, spoken idiomatically, are different sides to the same coin.

III. The Emergence of Disciplinary Cultures in the Modern Research University

My book accordingly aims at elucidating a middle ground – a meso-level view of science (see also Schweber 2006) between the macroscopic perspective of institutional sociology and the microscopic view of laboratory studies in STS. The concept of disciplinary cultures that I want to introduce helps focusing on this meso-level of disciplinary formation. It thereby enables viewing relevant processes somewhere between the abstract level of formal organization and the local level of material-epistemic practices. As I will illustrate, many of the now seemingly objective descriptions of

---

25 Surprisingly, queries for "scientific" or "research culture/s" (in the singular *and* plural) in the current *Handbook of Science and Technology Studies* total up to only ten mentions. That is an almost negligible figure compared to the number of "discipline/s" used in the text (see note 19 above).

medical science emerged from very specific institutions, research groups or laboratories. Overall, it can be said that disciplinary cultures received special significance with the emergence of modern science. Before that, the identity of a discipline was mainly determined by a body of philosophical knowledge, as noted above. In a classic account, Stichweh argues that modern disciplines emerged (in Germany) in a transitional period between the mid-eighteenth and the start of the nineteenth century (Stichweh 1992, 1984, see also Weingart 2010). During this process, the pursuit of science was relocated from the academy into the university, and disciplines developed from being classifications for epistemic subjects into social organizations or *scientific communities*. Before the nineteenth century, Stichweh shows, "the history of the term *disciplina* was closely linked to the history of the term *doctrina*" (1992: 4). In other words, disciplines were the context of learning in which students received the recorded doctrines, the teaching of a systematic set of philosophical knowledge.

In this respect, disciplines were not yet endowed with a specific social function, but "served as repositories of certified knowledge" (Weingart 2010: 4). In this configuration, knowledge was purely theoretical, and the cultural features focused on teaching and learning exclusively (Stichweh 1994b). Even in the higher faculties of law, medicine and theology, disciplinary knowledge neither instructed practice nor did it encourage scientific innovation, but only granted the graduating student the right to practice the corresponding profession because of scholarly credentials. As the sociologist Stephen Turner notes: "the key to academic culture was disputations – over the received texts" (2017: 15). Institutionally, the doctrines of *disciplina* were organized in the hierarchical structure of the medieval and early modern university. This structure was determined by the epistemic status of the different branches of knowledge – with the lower philosophical faculty and its propaedeutic teachings in the liberal arts as the basis for the higher faculties.[26]

Prior to the development of modern science, the university thus primarily constituted a place for scholarly and vocational training. Academic discourse happened mainly in the academies and learned societies, which were also responsible for the advancement of scientific knowledge. Their operational radius accordingly comprised mainly the natural and mathe-

---

26 Therefore, students of medicine had to first master "undergraduate" courses in the philosophical faculty before moving on to pursue a doctorate in medicine through education in a curriculum that contained specifically medical subjects like anatomy and physiology.

matical sciences.[27] The faculties of law, theology and medicine were generally excluded – and physicians, if they were a part, only partook in their capacity as natural researchers. Stichweh accordingly sees academies in this period characterized by three main features: The small number of personnel appeared to enable the conducting of "meaningful scientific work"; academies reflected the beginnings of the modern concept of science, which was oriented on the disciplines of the philosophical faculty; and the limitation of these institutional structures offered the opportunity to see and formulate an idea of *research* as a category that "distinguished the included from the excluded sciences", i.e., the natural sciences and mathematics from law, theology and medicine (1984: 67).

The cultural attributes of academies were also differentiated from those attributes central to university teaching and learning. An important feature of academies was that they defined "rules of discourse" for participation in scientific activities. Most prominently, institutions like the British Royal Society and the Prussian Academy of Science adopted the "practice of experimental proof" in the early eighteenth century, so that "topics that were part of the tradition of disputation and not subject to experimental evidence were excluded" (Turner 2017: 17, see also Shapin 2012: 89–116). According to Stichweh, such rules then became attributes of the modern university because of a "factual exodus of science out of the academy" at the end of the eighteenth century (1984: 69).

With the complex changes that (German) society underwent at the turn from the eighteenth to the nineteenth century, new social roles and demands for knowledge emerged. To educate the recruits to fill these new professional positions it required a high number of schoolteachers, who, in turn, had to be trained academically (McClelland 1980). Consequently, secondary education could no longer depend on the institutional authority of the family. Relocated to Gymnasia and *Realschulen*, it now rested on the epistemic certainty of the subjects that were taught and on their association with scientific knowledge. In the universities, this led to what Stichweh calls a "functional association between education and science" (ibid: 79). At the same time, scientific knowledge grew steadfast and fragmented, demanding criteria for its selective handling, and, because of its increasing mathematization, became more abstract and specialized (Weingart 2010: 5f.).

---

27 A historic-philological class was later added in Germany, but not in other European countries (Stichweh 1984: 68).

Under these conditions, the undifferentiated approach to scientific knowledge of the academies increasingly became unsustainable. Tending to all the areas of science, as it was now demanded by society, required a differentiated approach to academic subject areas. But the members of the academy were mostly private and not professional researchers; and their small number no longer provided the necessary labor forces for producing and transmitting knowledge in the different disciplinary fields. With the creation of new professions associated with secondary and university education, however, and the corresponding organizational growth of the university, the institution provided a combination of academic role structures and disciplinary categorizations, from which scientific careers could develop to accommodate the "different, quite heterogeneous, disciplines with their specific 'cultures' and the pursuit of research in the modern sense" (Weingart 2010: 7, see also Stichweh 1984: 87). As a result – and this is a common theme uniting sociological research on science since Kuhn – the cognitive differentiation and diversification of scientific knowledge could now rely on the organizational structure of the academic disciplines in the university for recruitment, bringing rules that defined the conduct of scientific activities into the institution, which replaced the traditional definition of disciplines as places of *doctrina*.[28] The teaching in universities now primarily comprised the transmission of these cultural properties instead of only teaching and learning the philosophical knowledge of a subject area. Stichweh refers to this change as the "dogmatization" of "scientific knowledge bases which are not dogmatical in themselves" (Stichweh 1994b: 191). Stated differently, the philosophical basis of a discipline was replaced with a set of "methods" or "practices" that were characteristic for the production of knowledge in a particular area. As Turner aptly concludes, disciplines now gained legitimacy "as the locus and guardian of specific competences and bodies of knowledge shared with others trained in the same discipline" (Turner 2017: 17).

IV. Academic Tribes and Disciplinary Territories

How can a systematic account of disciplinary culture be formulated in front of this historical genealogy? The aim is to provide a concept of

---

28 In this context, Stichweh speaks of "an exchange of functions", so that universities became places of research, while academies become refuges for learnedness (1984: 73).

disciplinarity that lies somewhere between the sociology of science and STS laboratory studies. I will draw on anthropological views of academic disciplines to develop this account. Already the American cultural anthropologist Clifford Geertz suggested an ethnographic look at disciplines in his book *Local Knowledge*, thereby anticipating my aim of finding a compromise between formal structure and local practice (Geertz 1983). He presented the prospect that such an analysis would reveal the different intellectual, political and moral relationships of members of a scientific community to each other and to the larger societal context; that it would bring to light the career structures and modes of socialization specific to individual disciplines; and that, moreover, "the vocabularies in which the various disciplines talk about themselves to themselves" could provide access "to the sort of mentalities at work in them" (1983: 157).

British higher education scholars Tony Becher and Paul Trowler have brought an anthropological perspective to bear on a systematic investigation of academic disciplines in their book *Academic Tribes and Territories* (2001). Based on extensive data from inquiries into fields in the humanities, social and natural sciences they argue that the knowledge structures of different disciplines ("territories") lead to the formation of specific disciplinary cultures ("tribes"). This means that the general behavior and the values of members constituting such cultures are formed by the practices, which they use to tend to their territory: "the ways in which academics engage with their subject matter, and the narratives they develop about this, are important structural factors in the formation of disciplinary cultures" (Becher/Trowler 2001: 23).

They develop a matrix that allows classifying disciplines into different categories. It relates epistemological properties of research areas with specific social aspects of disciplinary culture. Very briefly put, depending on whether the task of a group of researchers comprises working on "hard" or "soft" and "pure" or "applied" knowledge territories – e.g., whether that work concerns abstract and universal laws of the natural world or particular insights into the social world; and whether that knowledge is meant simply to explain or instead to inform social practices and professions – the resulting cultures can be categorized as being either "convergent" or "divergent" and "urban" or "rural", i.e., as tightly knit with lively exchange between members, and in which most researchers tend to the same or similar objects, or communities where members tend to different knowledge areas and have less interaction than in tightly knit communities. (Becher/Trowler 2001: 35ff., 183ff.).

What is crucial to my argument is that the authors go beyond Kuhn's notion of homogenous paradigms and scientific communities as well as beyond the sociology of scientific disciplines' formal dimensions of organizing science. Very much in the vein of Geertz (and of works in STS), they show how cultures of disciplines vary empirically regarding, e.g., career structures, publication practices or scientific standards.

> "In particular, the examination of the cognitive and social aspects of intellectual inquiry has highlighted a remarkable diversity in the activities that go to make up the academic enterprise. Knowledge areas, professional networks and individual career patterns can be classified, and operationally distinguished one from another, in a multiplicity of different ways" (Becher/Trwoler 2001: 194).

Put differently, Becher and Trowler identify for academic disciplines what scholars in STS identified for cultures of research – they constitute a vast landscape of heterogeneous fields with different approaches and social constitutions. However, by adhering to the concept of disciplines, the authors preserve part of the institutional perspective. For them, beyond the informal "patchwork[s] of overlapping groups, networks, and communities of practice" (Hackett et al. 2017: 739), which are characteristic of many works in STS, still lies a more formal dimension of organizing science. This provides an angle to incorporate theories about research cultures with those about the social institutions of science.

V. *Disciplines as Political Institutions*

Taking the broader perspective of culture, as I argued in the introduction, has the benefit of understanding science as the discursive and symbolic products of actors and of being able to historicize the idea of cultural formation. In the next two chapters, I set out to demonstrate how local cultures established and influence formal structures of science in Germany. Cultures, according to Becher and Trowler, can be defined as "sets of taken-for-granted values, attitudes and ways of behaving, which are articulated through and reinforced by recurrent practices among a group of people in a given context" (2001: 23). However, in their book, Becher and Trowler still assume the existence of an "epistemological core" as deterministic of the cultural characteristics of disciplines (see also Trowler 2014). Like Kuhn's paradigms, the essential link between a scientific epistemology and the social factors in disciplinary cultures, i.e., the norms, values and trajectories that form the basis to research work, is incompatible with the idea of science as cultural space. As Shapin notes, science constitutes "a diverse set of cultural practices, which may not have common methods, conventions or concepts, or at least common features to distinguish them from 'non-science' or common culture" (Shapin 1992: 346). The integration of these diverse cultural elements, as Harris (2005) argues, happens through reference to the "supercategory" science.

The form of essentialism implied in *Academic Tribes and Territories* can be avoided by complementing the idea of disciplinary cultures with a position like that of Pierre Bourdieu's *habitus*. Fundamentally, *habitus* describes "systems of durable, transposable dispositions [...], principles which generate and organize practices and representations that can be objectively adopted to their outcomes without presupposing a conscious aiming at ends or an express mastery of the operations necessary to attain them" (Bourdieu 1990: 53). It means that the possibilities of acting are not predetermined by explicit rules, which stem from overarching epistemic conditions like those given by knowledge areas nor are they simply determined by the local socio-material research settings. Instead, the notion of disciplinary cultures historicizes the possibilities for such actions. They are generated by immersion in the *tradition* of a disciplinary culture, through the "embodiment" of its history as the collective practice of pursuing science. *Habitus* "ensures the active presence of past experiences, which, deposited in each organism in the form of schemes of perception, thought and action, tend to guarantee the 'correctness' of practices and their constancy over time, more reliably than all formal rules and explicit norms" (Bourdieu 1990: 54).

What could be called a disciplinary *habitus*, therefore, incorporates "ways of knowing" and acting (Pickstone 2000), i.e., different forms of tacit (and explicit) knowledge coming from different scholarly traditions that students acquire through socialization into a specific disciplinary culture (Becher/Trowler 2001: 44ff.).[29] "Culture is both enacted and constructed," Becher and Trowler note, "played out according to structurally-provided scripts as well as changed during that process" (Becher/Trowler 2001: 24).

---

29 The past exemplars that determine Kuhn's paradigms, in contrast, are the express basis for consciously deriving rules to guide scientific activity. Becher and Trawler speak of "folkloric discourses and codes of practice and convention" and list elements, such as tacit and explicit knowledge, a special language, and practical, methodological, or theoretical devices commonly employed, which make up the values, attitudes and ways of behaving within a respective field (Becher/Trowler 2001: 48).

In a Foucauldian sense, moreover, one could also say that scholars are *disciplined* into programs for specific ways of scientific action that become embodied as routine techniques and patterns of cognition and communication (Lenoir 1997: 47ff.).[30] Being part of a disciplinary community therefore comes with "a sense of identity and personal commitment" that provides a cultural frame determining much of one's everyday life (Becher/Trowler 2001: 47, see also Knorr Cetina 1999: 129f.). Having defined being part of a disciplinary culture through the embodiment of the different schemas of perception, thought and action, members of a discipline also embody a specific way of life, a "scientific life" (Shapin 2008), something that actors strive to maintain and defend.

If disciplines sustain specific ways of scientific life, it is no far leap to interpret them also as institutions that combine the intellectual interests of researchers with their social and political conditions. Taking "either a political economy or a cultural approach" (Schweber 2008: 15), some social historians of science therefore argue that scientific institutions like disciplines are formed at the intersection where the collective interests of science meet with the individual interests of researchers. In his classic institutional history *From Medical Chemistry to Biochemistry*, Robert Kohler introduces disciplines as "political institutions that demarcate areas of academic territory, allocate the privileges and responsibilities of expertise, and structure claims to resources" (Kohler 1982: 1, see also Kohler 1979: 28). He was taking his cues from the American historian Charles Rosenberg, who maintained that a scientific life needs to be regarded as a "compromise" between the "sometimes consistent and sometimes conflicting demands" of intellectual work in a discipline "and the particular conditions of an individual's employment" (Rosenberg 1997: 230). In other words, it is vital to not only look at the intellectual programs of researchers, but also at the institutional context in which they were articulated in order to understand their social significance for the development of science (e.g., Schweber 2008). "The totality of any discipline or profession", Rosenberg explains, "must be seen as a series of parallel intellectual activities being carried on in a variety of social contexts. Such rubrics as the humanities,

---

30 Another way of putting it – also with Foucauldian connotations – would be to invoke the idea of "epistemic virtues" at the heart of Lorraine Daston's and Peter Galison's book *Objectivity* (2010). Especially the virtue of "trained judgement", which they portray as emerging in the mid- to late-nineteenth century is compatible with the disciplinary developments that interest me, since it is based on modes of instruction, "in which students internalized and calibrated standards for seeing, judging, evaluating, and arguing" (ibid: 327).

life sciences, or social sciences mask diversity as much as they imply unity" (Rosenberg 1997: 230).

This model of disciplines is furthermore compatible with the idea of a scientific field, the complementary concept to Bourdieu's *habitus* (Lenoir 1997: 52f.). For Bourdieu, a field is a relational analytical concept in which actors struggle over different forms of capital (symbolic, cultural, political etc.) (Bourdieu/Wacquant 1992: 97). While a field as such is unobservable (and we cannot equate disciplines with fields), the advantage of the field perspective is that we can understand the struggles going on inside of them in relation to a range of heterogeneous elements in society not immediately visible as connected to science. In concrete terms, through the concept of a field, knowledge production in a disciplinary context can be seen as linked to practical requirements of the state and administration, or to cultural and ideological frames in society, or to the industry both in terms of economic interests and as a material prerequisite for providing research technologies and lab equipment (Lenoir 1997: 239ff.). The practices of scientific actors thus become embedded in a web of social relations that determine their position within the field. The relevance of this perspective for my study is that disciplinary identity is not formed by the subject matter of a science, by specific epistemologies or by corresponding practices and methods, but by the relation of these to the expectations of stakeholders and other areas of society.[31]

Bourdieu defines the scientific field as a "locus of competitive struggle, in which the specific issue at stake is the monopoly of scientific authority" or "the monopoly over scientific competence, in the sense of a particular agent's socially recognized capacity to speak and act legitimately [...] in scientific matters" (Bourdieu 1975: 19). However, scientific competence or the capacity to speak and act legitimately in matters of science is not only a product of scientific actors' epistemic endeavors. Instead, the intellectual pursuits are themselves a resource in the struggle to acquire the cultural capital, with which one can bargain for the necessary resources to pursue further scientific projects. This view deliberately blurs the distinction between a technical and political side of scientific knowledge production: "The political struggle to dominate resources is inseparable from the

---

31 I will show especially in the case of medical and biological sciences in the early-twentieth century USA (chapter 5) that their research practices as well as their institutional organization became virtually indistinguishable. The only distinguishing factor that remained was how actors in these fields related their academic work to social demands and expectations.

cognitive enterprise of defining what constitutes legitimate, authorized science" (Lenoir 1997: 52).[32] From this perspective, ideas, methods or techniques receive primacy as *cultural* items over their implied *intellectual* meaning. They can be discursively mobilized as a way for individuals and groups to politically maintain their status and identity within the social system of science. Thus, the technical aspects of scientific ideas are inseparable from their political function in the context of institution-building: "Ideas and research programs are professional strategies and one cannot separate their intellectual and political aspects" (Kohler 1982: 214, see also Kohler 1979: 56f.).[33]

VI. Disciplinary Boundary and Identity Work

The political struggles over resources and influences as well as the interlinking of professional and social interests can be conceptualized as disciplinary *boundary work* (Gieryn 1995, 1999) and *identity work* (Kaldewey 2013). Disciplines, I want to accordingly propose, are institutions that are constantly in flux, their identities permanently reproduced and renegotiated according to the changing social and scientific contexts. As Kohler

---

32 After his discussion of Bourdieu in his cultural theory of disciplines, historian Timothy Lenoir, however, introduces a problematic distinction between "research programs" and "disciplinary programs" (1997: 53ff.). Research programs constitute the problem-oriented instrumental practices akin to those that make up research cultures; disciplinary programs, in contrast, operate on the institutional level of science, where "scientific entrepreneurs" with managerial skill promote the research work in a political economy to build the according institutions. But by separating "the labor and political work struggles involved in research work form the quite different politics and work of discipline building" (ibid: 53), Lenoir implies that the latter is not represented in the former. My point is precisely that the choice of techniques, methods and practices for scientific work are always also entangled with social and cultural values and ideals. In other words, while Lenoir implies an image of scientists of problem-solving lab drones, who's work requires being translated into cultural products that can be understood by society, I want to suggest that all researchers are always scientific practitioners and managers of scientific identity.

33 Knorr Cetina maintains, in contrast, that "those amalgams of arrangements and mechanisms" which make up epistemic cultures were simply "bonded through affinity, necessity, and historical coincidence" (1999: 1, see also Knorr Cetina/Reichmann 2015: 873). This assumption misses the central point, however, that the cultural frames, which define the actions of a given group of researchers, as well as the objects they are committed to, emerged over time.

makes clear right at the outset of his book, disciplines "are creatures of history and reflect human habits and preferences, not a fixed order of nature" (Kohler 1982: 1). Or as Gieryn warns readers, "The analytical danger is to reify the cultural space of science into something so stable, so 'structural', or 'institutionalized', that the significance of episodic reproductions in boundary-work is lost altogether" (Gieryn 1995: 420). In practices of discursive demarcation, actors continuously defend the status and relevance of their discipline in the institutional context of science. In their papers, pamphlets and speeches, they constantly readjust their practical work to jurisdictional claims over intellectual and societal problems. These discourses are not merely "epiphenomena" of the competition between disciplines, but important aspects through which disciplines form their social, moral and intellectual orders in the first place (Amsterdamska 2005: 46).

Olga Amsterdamska (2005) impressively examines the strategic use of ideas and methods for epidemiological discipline-building, drawing on the conceptual frame of boundary-work. She uses the approach to illuminate the "internal" border-drawing that designates "the place and the status of a specific discipline" (ibid: 20). Epidemiologists distinguished their pursuit from that of bacteriology and other medical sciences in the early-twentieth century to argue for its academic autonomy on the one hand, but also from statistics in order to claim its scientific status as opposed to being simply an instrument for public health officials on the other. In the process, academic epidemiologists employed different devices of science, such as laboratory experiment, biostatistical analysis or field observation, framing them as part of their disciplinary identity. In the interwar period, for example, actors distinguished the epidemiological concept of disease from the idea of "disease that was an object of a clinical or bacteriological investigation", in order to subject it to their statistical forms of explanation, calling for cognitive and institutional autonomy (ibid: 32). But after World War II, epidemiologists no longer contrasted the "logic of statistical inference" with the "logic of experimentation" but instead now framed statistics as a means to overcome the "possible shortcomings of [experimental] research" (ibid: 43). Such discursive boundary-drawing, as Amsterdamska emphasizes, are mainly directed at peers, "to the actual practitioners who are thus being reminded both of the scientific nature of their endeavor and of their membership in a select and distinctive community" (ibid: 46).

As research on identity work, more generally, has shown, scientific identity is constructed not only in relation to scientific peers. It is rather an interplay of scientific self-attributions and of negotiations over the role of science opposed to societal attributions and expectations (Kaldewey 2013:

107, Schauz 2020: 22). Thereby, identity work contributes to remapping the public image of science in accordance with expectations and desires of different non-scientific actors just as much as it reorganizes intra-science relations. Disciplinary identity can thus be seen to emerge from the tension between work understood as free and only devoted to scientific truth as well as the simultaneous expectation of its social utility. Discursive identity work means exploring how actors in their communications claimed specific research techniques, methods, concepts or styles as professional markers and how they also distinguished them from other professional groups by drawing cultural boundaries. Disciplinary boundary work is thus always simultaneously an act of exclusion and inclusion. Moreover, they used these devices to position their actions between the often local social and economic conditions of their professional work and the intellectual and structural contexts of science. For example, discarding the empirical method of clinical medicine in favor laboratory practices is at the same time a strategy to stake off professional turf within medical science, just as much as it is a symbol for committing to the general ideology of cultural progress through science.

Instances of disciplinary identity work are visible in actors of the early-twentieth century US university landscape. As Rosenberg, for example, shows, scientists who held leading positions in research stations or departments at the time acted in a political and scientific double role, which he calls "scientist-entrepreneurs" or "research-entrepreneurs" (Rosenberg 1997: 159, see also Kohler 1982: 5, Lenoir 1997: 46). Their characteristic feature was, according to Rosenberg, that in order to secure the institutional viability of their disciplines, they mediated between the world of science on the one hand and the world of social and economic expectations of a certain group of clients on the other (e.g., governments, businesses, public institutions). "The successful research-entrepreneur had to not only tailor a research policy to the needs of his lay constituency, but still remain aware of professional values and realities" (Rosenberg 1997: 159). In exchange for the institutionally secured possibility to pursue research freely, agrarian scientists, for instance, began to equip the identity of their discipline with specific service functions, such as the promise to find ways to maximize yield or breed productive strains of crop. Shapin reconstructed forms of identity work using the example of the Biotech-Boom in the 1970s and 1980s, where scientists established remarkable businesses with the help of venture capital. Consequently, a figure rose to prominence that is defined by embodying the tension between science and social contexts: "They had one foot in the making of knowledge and the other in the making of artifacts, services, and, ultimately, money" (Shapin 2008: 210).

Next to actions of research, i.e., the actual production of scientific knowledge, working in an institution like a discipline always also entails a form of praxis that relates research to different social contexts. In their quotidian practices, scientists not only play the role of problem-solving lab drones, but also contribute to the (self-)depictions of disciplines and research cultures, which often also include promises of utility and relevance that legitimize their research practices in front of a broader public and stakeholders in society. Accordingly, discipline specific socialization, or the acquisition of a disciplinary *habitus*, comprises, next to initiation into a community's ways of knowing and acting, that students already learn how their prospective academic work is linked to expectations of services, which are often already expressed in the descriptions of study programs at universities.[34] Thus, looking through the analytical lens of disciplinary identity has the advantage of transforming the sociological issue of science's dis-/unity into an empirical question of discursive boundary and identity work (Kaldewey 2013: 107). In what follows, I will show that one can neither speak of a clear organizational unity nor of a fragmented field, but that the different research cultures of medical science are held together by the basic concepts that characterize the discipline as at the same time an intellectual and political endeavor.

---

34 See for example the promises of utility and social relevance in the self-description of the BA-program "Molecular Biomedicine" at the University of Bonn: https://www.uni-bonn.de/de/studium/studienangebot/studiengaenge-a-z/molekulare-biomedizin-bsc (accessed July 29th, 2021).

3. The Birth of a Modern Discipline – Medicine as *Wissenschaft* in German Romanticism

The categorization that was first used to classify medicine as a modern academic discipline was "medicine as *Wissenschaft*" (Reil 1804, 1910, Schelling 1805). The key concept gained popularity during the founding of the University of Berlin in 1809/10. Berlin's first university (the precursor to today's Humboldt University) acts as a paragon of the modern research university, established in the spirit of Romantic educational reform associated with the names Wilhelm von Humboldt, Johann Gottlieb Fichte and Friedrich von Schleiermacher (see Schelsky 1971, Tenorth 2012). For the idea of science, the Age of Romanticism constituted a considerable breach with the preceding Enlightenment utilitarianism. Enlighteners followed an ideology of social progress, which valued knowledge mostly for its usefulness. Effectively, this resulted in the levelling of knowledge from university-educated people and "amateurs" towards practical goals. For actors that identified with academic qualities, this posed a great threat to their professional identity. Toward the end of the eighteenth century, therefore, circles of academically learned natural researchers began defending their trade. They distinguished more clearly between theoretical and practical areas of scientific knowledge to separate their work from immediate utility and requirements of the state and society (Phillips 2012). In the course, a new concept emerged: *Wissenschaft*; the idea of a pure form of academic science devoid of any immediate concerns for usefulness. The term had become widely used by the turn to the nineteenth century and stood for the systematic unity of scientific knowledge, which preceded all practical interests (Kaldewey 2013: 283, Stichweh 2007: 213f.).

The concept of *Wissenschaft* became a central item in arguments, which stated that science had to be pursued entirely for its own sake. As I will explain further down, the use of *Wissenschaft* in the singular deviated from common references to the *Wissenschaften*, or "sciences" in the plural, as the broad denominator for all kinds of knowledge. In contrast to the English term "science", which describes the natural (and technical) sciences more narrowly, the word "*Wissenschaft*" meant the unity of all academic knowledge taught and pursued at the university (including philosophy and the humanities).[35] Engagement with *Wissenschaft*, Romantics argued, would not only provide practitioners with a thorough understanding of natural and cultural phenomena; it would also contribute to the *Bildung* – understood as both formation *and* education – of a person's character, making him (higher education was restricted to men in the early nineteenth century) naturally prone to contribute to the common good of society and to cultural progress. However, in the case of the natural sciences, the condition was that nature had to be studied in its entirety and as a unity,[36] and not only in aspects that made it suitable for application, as the Enlightenment knowledge systems proposed. "Practical men who studied practical problems knew only bits and pieces of nature; only the learned man knew nature as a whole" (Phillips 2012: 90).

For members of the medical elite, learnedness constituted a crucial marker of their professional identity. From the late Middle Ages until the Age of Enlightenment, the traditional professions of law, theology and medicine were based on the qualities that came with higher education. Symbolized in erudition, Latinity, an academic character and lifestyle, these qualities "surrounded the local practitioner with an aura of honorific distinction, before which considerations of function or social utility paled" (Turner 1980: 108, see also Phillips 2012: 27–39). For a Doctor of Medicine, the ability to practice derived more or less automatically from his identity as a scholar, from his membership in an academic community – certified by his university degree – that possessed a broad knowledge of the philosophical and medical tradition (in contrast to the clinical proficiency required today). But the later eighteenth century brought what R. Steven Turner has aptly characterized as a shift from an emphasis on "learned expertise" to "functional expertise" (1980: 109). This shift sent shockwaves through the university world, forcing academic researchers to redefine their highly theoretical pursuits in face of public demands for applicability. Works in the social history of medicine have shown how the traditional image of the academic physician as a learned man (there were also no women doctors at the time) came under pressure in the eighteenth century, since the Enlightenment's ideology valued knowledge, instead of for its academic qualities, primarily for its practical utility and benefit for

---

35 For issues when translating *Wissenschaft* into English see Phillips (2012: 3–6, 2015).

36 What this exactly meant in the context of medicine will become apparent in this chapter.

social progress (e.g., Frevert 1984, Huerkamp 1985, Lindemann 1996, see also Turner 1980).

The explanations offered by the literature, however, are predicated on modern ideas of professionalism (Broman 1996). Accordingly, academically trained physicians are portrayed as having organized themselves so that they could make exclusive jurisdictional claims to healing practices and expulse non-academic medical services from the marketplace.[37] Academic science, some historians argue, served mainly as an emblem, which distinguished the learned physician from the wide range of craft medicine practitioners, such as surgeons, barbers, midwives or apothecaries. Other authors have critiqued that this view casts an anachronistic image of early modern physicians and of early modern professions more generally (Broman 1996: 4ff., Lindemann 1996: 168f., 372f.). It reduces physicians' identities to practical qualities – something that does not sit well with historical ideas of medicine – although they thought of themselves in the main part as members of the learned estate and only secondarily referred to their identity as healers. What, then, happened to the academic identity of physicians during and after the Enlightenment?

Historian Thomas Broman (1996) has moved explanations a step further. He notes how, drawn between the demands of the idea of "pure science", introduced by the Romantic reformers, and the delivery of medicine to society, two occupations effectively came out of the medical profession: one tended to medical research in universities and the other concerned the practice of healing in local communities (Broman 1989, see also Broman 1996: 161). As academic medicine was transforming into the experimental study of organic nature on the one side, and the clinical aspect of medicine was evolving on the other, the identities of the physician as academic scholars *and* as practical healers were becoming increasingly incompatible (ibid: 48). Consequently, Broman argues, a new type of medical professor developed, with a self-conception that distinguished him (again, only men in the early-nineteenth century) from former ideas of the physician, in that they "removed themselves as far as possible from [medical] practice" (ibid: 51). These new professors subsequently began organizing their work towards ends that would later become the laboratory research of animal morphology, Broman argues.

---

37 For historian Thomas Broman, this is an anachronistic argument. Such "claims about early modern physicians arise from the same problem: the inappropriateness of applying criteria of modern professionalism to its early modern version" (Broman 1996: 6).

For many authors writing about German science and medicine in the late eighteenth and early nineteenth century, this development marks the starting point for the purported change from a medical to a biological identity of full-time researchers working in the medical faculty. The idea is that, while physicians outside the faculty acquired a primarily practical identity, those that remained in the university, since they factually cut their ties to medical practice, must have consequently become pure researchers in biological areas. From this standpoint, however, portrayals of the scientific developments in academic medicine at the time are predetermined by our current views of biology. In short, the scientific developments in medicine are depicted as the prelude to the biological developments that came later in the century. But the modern academic discipline of biology was still in its infancy at that point and largely characterized by eighteenth-century approaches in natural history and the tradition of taxonomic practices in botany and zoology. Morphological studies, which Borman refers to, were pursued as part of the *medical* faculty and research community (Nyhart 1995). How did these new professors of medicine, who devoted their professional life entirely to research, maintain their intimate ties to medical institutions? How were they able to also retain the right to practice and teach under the roof of the medical faculty? And how were these actors, with an interest in understanding living nature rather than in the practice of healing, furthermore able to sustain their professional trajectories if no institutions for laboratory research in biology existed at the time?

My answer to the questions above takes on the perspective of medicine as a genuine academic discipline. The general concept of disciplines that emerged with the modern research university was that of the unity of research and teaching (Stichweh 1994b). Even though practitioners henceforth devoted themselves to biological questions in research, as will become apparent, they were nevertheless still obliged to teach medical students. Against the arguments in the literature, I argue that, although henceforth devoted to laboratory research on phenomena of organic nature, these actors retained their medical identity in order to not jeopardize their newfound professional trajectories, i.e., access to future recruits that could continue their laboratory culture of medical science. Chairs in biology were not installed until the mid-nineteenth century, meaning that no study curriculum yet existed that taught experimental research to understand biological phenomena. Even the subsequent development of biology as a laboratory science depended on the institutional basis laid by academic medicine at the start of the century (Nyhart 1995).

Therefore, instead of a clear separation between the institutions of medical practice and laboratory research, between profession and science, I want to show how the discipline of medicine functioned doubly: it provided the opportunity for immersion into an intellectual culture seen as required for both medical practitioners *and* researchers. The idea of an academic discipline that was formed under the rubric of medicine as *Wissenschaft* simultaneously satisfied the requirements of the scientific community for intellectual autonomy and the interests of the state for educating practitioners that provided health care. Rather than oppose academic ideals with state ideals of practical utility, the concept of medicine as *Wissenschaft* opened a conceptual space in which different existing institutions of the university and of medicine came together to form the modern institution of education in the natural sciences for physicians. In a sense, the discipline was a territory for two future tribes (biology and medicine) or sustained an academic *habitus* that was presented as suitable for both medical education and laboratory practice. Crucial to this early development was that actors began pressing for laboratory research as fundamental for future physicians, applying the Romantic arguments of character formation and the need for a holistic understanding of nature. In a diachronic perspective, this analysis can help explain why medical students ever since are required to take intensive training in laboratory courses and it can also indicate why basic laboratory research is so tightly linked to ideas of biomedicine today.

In this chapter, I want to reconstruct the conceptual and institutional developments of academic medicine in the context of Berlin's university founding. For this purpose, I will be concentrating on texts by Johann Christian Reil on the organization of medical education in Berlin. Reil, initially physician and professor of medicine at the University of Halle, is a key player because he served as advisor to Humboldt during the academic reforms of Prussia and was later appointed as professor to the new University of Berlin (Broman 1996: 183, see also 1989: 46f.). He was also an important protagonist to prominently employ the new concept of medicine as *Wissenschaft* in his texts (Reil 1804, 1910). Using this category, Reil conceptually differentiated between theoretical and practical areas in medicine to make medical science a subject pursued purely for its own sake. He furthermore proposed reorganizing existing academic medical institutions according to the principles of Romantic science, thereby opening a conceptual and institutional space into which medicine as a scientific discipline could be inserted.

In sum, the notion of medicine as *Wissenschaft* allowed academic physicians to define their professional identity as distant from actual medical practice, while simultaneously framing their research culture as foundational for the practice of medicine. To provide modern medical science with a distinct disciplinary culture within the academic system, moreover, actors in medicine reinvented physiology to make it the core of medical science's research culture. In the process, the pre- and early modern idea of physiology as comprising theoretical doctrines about organic nature was turned into a practical science, which appropriated practices traditionally associated with anatomy (Cunningham 2002, 2003). Structurally, a relationship to the medical faculty was retained by framing an immersion in these practices as a requirement for the academically trained physician.

I will first try to give a brief overview of the institutional *status quo* prior to the opening of Berlin's university. Then I want to reflect on the conceptual innovation "medicine as *Wissenschaft*". Placing Reil's ideas in the wider context of scientific concepts as well as the existing institutions of academic medicine (in Berlin), I demonstrate how he reorganized them to argue for the need of a medical science discipline. I ask how it is distinguished from precursor concepts and evaluate its institutional ramifications for academic medicine.

I. Medicine Between Art and Learnedness – The Conceptual Background

This section and the next are devoted to providing the necessary context for understanding the conceptual and institutional innovations that occurred at the start of the nineteenth century. Naturally, what Reil and his conspirators proposed was not constructed into a vacuum. Rather, in important instances they made use of the existing institutions and conceptions and transformed their meanings, next to introducing genuinely novel concepts. To give a thorough background would require writing a book of its own. Here, I can only provide a quick pass-through of pinnacle events and changes from the classic period until early modernity. My purpose is to, in very broad strokes, sketch major shifts in conceptual relations between medical theory and practice in order to appreciate the ingenuity of the categorical changes introduced by Reil and the Romantic reformers.

Since Greek antiquity, beginning with Hippocrates (2012), the defining marker of medicine had been the concept of "art" or *techne* (table 3.1). In the Classical world, the term *techne* comprised a large spectrum of activities that ranged from rhetoric to carpentry. The basic tenet of the arts was that their results were deliberate and artificial products, which "would not have existed without the intervention of a technician, a practitioner of techne" (Schatzberg 2018: 18). Greek society, therefore, made no explicit distinction between occupations that were highly theoretical or predominantly practical. But the concept of *techne* did imply a relationship between theory and practice that was determined by the fact that the arts required *logos*, rational thought about cause and effects (ibid: 20). It is therefore important to note that at its inception medicine was defined from its *practical* side, while its characterization from the *scientific* side is a decidedly modern phenomenon, picking up especially with the Romantic reformers. Before, however, as I will show further down, medicine would receive a composite academic identity, which in the eighteenth century would begin to be expressed in the vernacular terms of "science" and "art" (*Wissenschaft* and *Kunst*).

The Middle Ages witnessed the introduction of the concept of the "mechanical arts", which led to the distinction of artisanal from the scholarly activities of the "liberal arts" (ibid: 30–41). Since medicine came from a tradition of *techne*, and therefore fell outside of the range of Classical conceptions of either philosophy or politics, it was initially classified as a "mechanical art" in the emerging academic canon (ibid: 34, see also Amundsen 1979: 55ff., Bylebyl 1990: 30f., Kaldewey 2013: 327f.). Accordingly, to receive a place in the higher studies of the university, medical actors fought "to make the lowly and manual craft of medicine part of a properly instituted *studium generale*" (French 2003: 80). After Scholastic scholars rediscovered Aristotle's philosophy from Arabic translations in the twelfth and thirteenth century, the strategy involved framing the formerly only implicit theoretical part of the medical art as explicitly dependent on the study of nature; that is, particularly on Aristotle's natural philosophy (ibid: 107–113).

As a result, medicine received its identity as a learned subject, in which the Latin term *scientia* expressed its conformity with logic and philosophical reason and *ars* retained its identity as a practical art. In the process, however, the concept of medicine shed the practice of surgery, which had been an integral part of its ancient identity but conflicted with the idea of an intellectual enterprise due to the associations with manual labor (Amundsen 1979, see also Bylebyl 1990: 40). Since notions of production associated with the Greek term *techne* moved to the background, the "practical" side of the academic physician now not only became restricted to internal medicine (something that could be practiced in discourse, without the use of hands), but also superimposed with features of rational judgement and prudent behavior inherent to Aristotelian philosophy (Bylebyl 1990: 32–40). Until about the eighteenth century, according to medical historian Roger French, the physician therefore comprised the image of a "Learned and Rational Doctor", which primarily meant the possession of a great deal of knowledge of the ancients and of skills for arguing dialectically and philosophically (French 2003: 2). By that time, their identity of medieval learnedness had also become complemented with ideals of early modern gentility (ibid: 200ff., see also Huerkamp 1985: 34).

	medical theory	**medical practice**
400–200 BCE	*[logos]*	*techne*
12.–13. century	*scientia*	*ars*
17.–18. century	*Wissenschaft*	*Kunst*
	pure science	**applied science**

Table 3.1: Concepts for distinguishing between medical theory and practice in premodern times (from 400 BCE to c. 1800) (my depiction).

During the eighteenth century, medicine was talked about in connection with the terms "science" and "art". However, using these concepts, one did not draw a clear line between medicine's purely theoretical parts, on the one hand, and the practice of healing, on the other. Sciences and arts in the eighteenth century, as historian of technology Eric Schatzberg notes, "existed on a continuum defined by the purity of reason, with substantial overlap between the two extremes" (2018: 57, see also Phillips 2012: 35ff.). Accordingly, descriptions of medicine as a "healing" or "medicinal science" (*Heilwissenschaft* or *Arzneywissenschaft*), or as a "healing" or "medicinal art" (*Heilkunst* or *Arzneykunst*), were largely interchangeable before 1800.[38] The *Deutsche Encyclopädie*, for example, published in twenty-three volumes between 1778 and 1804 as a "dictionary of all arts and sciences", speaks of the "medicinal art [*Arzneykunst*]" as "a science [*Wissenschaft*]" that teaches how to preserve health and heal diseases (Höpfner 1778: 839). Therefore, in obvious Enlightenment fashion, all medical knowledge, whether theoretical or practical, was organized towards the end of healing. Consequently, the dictionary portrays the doctor as the individual who

---

38 Nevertheless, the difference in wording did tend to highlight either the theoretical or practical side, when used in conversation.

performs "the medicinal art [*Arzneykunst*]" and who must be versed in the "practical" just as much as in the "theoretical sciences [*Wissenschaften*] of medicine [*Arzneykunde*]" (ibid: 851).

The rise to popularity of *Wissenschaft* by 1800 introduced not only a clear distinction, but also a hierarchy between theoretical and practical knowledge. The term denoted the unified organization of scientific knowledge and made the study of natural phenomena the exclusive domain of academic research. While previously everybody who collected and contributed what today would be called "data" about the natural world could be a natural researcher,[39] recourse to *Wissenschaft*, as a unified science of nature, drew a clear boundary between university-educated and other "lay" natural researchers (Phillips 2012). Historian Denise Phillips demonstrates how the whole range of natural scientific academic practitioners in early nineteenth-century Germany pursued the aim of creating a "general natural science" (2012: 86). The term *Wissenschaft* serves today mostly as an epitome for the pure science ideal of the Prussian reformers, the ascent of the philosophical faculty within the university system, and as a path leading to *Bildung*. On a broader scale, as Phillips argues, the category was employed as a social project for protagonists, such as the actors of *Naturphilosophie*, to defend the scientific enterprise against usurpation by the functional ideology of the Enlightenment.

Since practical sciences proved highly popular well into the nineteenth century, the strategy of academics to defend their learned identity involved "separating theoretical from practical intellectual forums", which resulted in increasing the relevance for societies and media that devoted themselves exclusively to learned subjects (ibid: 89). As Phillips shows, the concept was therefore at the heart of the strategy of learned professionals to remove themselves from the responsibility for practice. "Once this new ideal of *Wissenschaft* rose to prominence," she notes, "older descriptions of the learned '*Wissenschaften und Künste*' came to seem quaint and dated […]. In the early nineteenth century, *Wissenschaft* finally shed its more expansive early modern meaning. It was no longer used to designate just 'knowledge' (both academic and nonacademic) in general; more important, it lost its

---

39 In a related vein, Stichweh (1994a: 59f.) has characterized the early-modern scientific system as allopoietic, i.e., the expansion of scientific knowledge by inclusion and indexing of things from the system's environment, instead of the construction of the scientific system via self-produced elements, e.g., epistemic objects or traces created in laboratory experiment (see also Hacking 1992, Rheinberger 1997).

early modern partner, the learned '*Künste*,' a term that also sometimes functioned as its synonym" (ibid: 98). Accordingly, now the idea of the university professor was to confer upon students the broad moral and intellectual education that leads to *Bildung* (Turner 1980: 127ff.). "By distinguishing between merely 'useful' and truly 'learned' knowledge," Phillips concludes, "elite *Naturforscher* neatly exempted themselves from thorny, complicated questions about their practical relevance" (2012: 113). In the case of medicine as *Wissenschaft*, the idea also implied an occupational separation – a division of labor that distinguished between the scientific and practical tasks of medicine.

II. The Institutional Environment in Prussia's Capital

The institutional context into which the reform plans and the new language of academic medicine was born was complex. The University of Berlin was founded into a landscape that already harbored a well-established system of medical education. Historian Arleen Tuchman (2000) has characterized the institutional environment that developed with the birth of the University of Berlin as a "confusing triangle". By this she is especially referring to the tensions that formed between the new medical faculty and the existing medical schools, especially the competition over resources, facilities and the general orientation of academic medicine. The landscape at the time comprised, first, the *Collegium Medico-Chirurgicum*, a practical training school for military and civilian medical personnel established in the early-eighteenth century, and later, the Pépinière, an elite military medical academy founded in 1795, as well as the Charité hospital (Hess 2010a, Tuchmann 2000). Medical doctors who began devoting their professional life mainly to research, and exempted themselves from practice, had to therefore make a strong case for establishing theoretical medicine as a research discipline. Despite the new classification of medicine as a purely academic pursuit, they had to nevertheless link their discipline to the predominating practical interests of the local medical community and the Prussian state. The idea of a medical research discipline that emerged from the concept of *Wissenschaft* was therefore not strictly anti-practical. Instead, it retained a strong bond to medical practice, although by arguing that only physicians trained under the pure science ideal will possess the professional and personal qualities for the adequate treatment of patients. Before moving on to important conceptual and institutional developments, I want to set the stage for my inquiry by briefly sketching the relationships between the different institutions that existed at the time.

Prior to the founding of the new university, medical education in Berlin was predetermined by Enlightenment thinking, especially by the military interests of the Prussian state. Under the reign of Friedrich Wilhelm I., who induced reforms in medical education in the early eighteenth century, the city first received an anatomical theater in 1713 for performing dissections and later, in 1725, saw the establishment of a *Collegium medico-chirurgicum* (Broman 1996: 53f., Tuchman 2000: 38f.). These practical medical schools, which could also be found in other German cities, were erected to rear a new caste of military and civilian medico-surgeons (Bonner 1995: 53ff.). The model of medical education they represented, was exemplary of how in the ideology of the Enlightenment knowledge was being combined and taught to be both systematic and useful. In the eighteenth century, "new practical sciences" developed inside and outside of academia to improve agriculture, forestry, mining and other trades. The aim was to increase the productivity of society and thereby foster state powers. Many formerly purely academic subjects thus became conjoined with topics from economy or the crafts, recasting the ancient distinction between theory and practice and thereby turning many learned teachings into useful arts and sciences (Phillips 2012: 35, see also Broman 1996: 46f.).

The new medical academies furthermore broke the monopoly that guilds held over surgical training and contributed to the rapprochement between medicine and surgery by transgressing their intellectual and disciplinary boundaries (Bonner 1995: 56ff.). Already in the Middle Ages, after its separation from academic medicine, and despite the common image of a lowly craft, some actors began employing arguments for the requirement of academic credentials for surgery in framing it as a learned and rational enterprise (Wallis 2018: 58f.). In the early modern German territories, elite surgeons exhibited "academic standards in their training and lifestyle", although maintaining "an identity of 'medical artisans'" (Rabier 2018: 83). Surgeons argued extensively for the scientific foundation of their craft, especially by appropriating for it the subject of anatomy. These precursory developments fed into the idea of the practical medical schools by, on the one hand, combining an academic curriculum with practical instruction and, on the other, educating practitioners in both internal medicine and surgery.

Universities tried to intercept these developments in the eighteenth century by also orienting themselves towards practical requirements, but they were generally no match for the new academies favored by rulers for their military relevance. Even though surgery had been the subject of lectures by the medical faculty before, universities also began offering clinical and theoretical surgery courses by the end of the century. "The old distinction", as medical historian Thomas Bonner observes, "between the 'medical surgery' of the university and the 'practical surgery' outside them was beginning to fade" (1995a: 58). As a result of the integration of theoretical and practical medical knowledge, the professional distinction between medicine and surgery turned into a disciplinary distinction within the same medical curriculum (Weisz 2006: 196–203). Additionally, an edict by the Prussian government later in 1825, which set completely new rules for medical licensing, effectively abolished the legal distinction between the practice of surgeons and academic doctors (Huerkamp 1985: 45–50, see also Turner 1980: 117–120).

Thus, the medical education system of the Enlightenment undermined the clear distinction of medicine into an academic science and a practical art. The *Collegium* in Berlin, for instance, had seven full professors and aimed at combining theoretical with practical teaching: "One could listen to lectures in anatomy, surgery, physiology, pathology, pharmacology, physics and mathematics, while attending the anatomical and surgical exercises in the anatomical theater" (Tuchman 2000: 38). Whereas everybody eligible for higher education could study at the institution, its express goal was to produce military surgeons, and most students were in fact enrolled in this track (Hess 2010a: 62, Tuchman 2000: 38). Students received a thorough education, comparable in quality to that at universities, but with a stronger emphasis on practical training. The only thing that distinguished them effectively was the lack of a doctoral degree. The *Collegium*'s faculty was comprised of court physicians, the leading surgeons and physicians of the military and further medical experts (some of which would later also become part of the medical faculty of Berlin's university). According to Volker Hess, "it thereby represented the medical elite of the capital" (Hess 2010a: 62). Next to the anatomical theatre, the school also had access to the Berlin Academy of Science's botanical garden and the chemical laboratory of the Court Apothecary – a luxury that distinguished it from the existing Prussian universities (Broman 1996: 53). Since the *Collegium* far surpassed any medical faculty in Prussia in both facilities and importance, Broman even argues that it acted as "a sort of shadow medical faculty" (ibid.).

Developments toward the end of the eighteenth century aggravated the situation of academic medicine even further. In 1795, Friedrich Wilhelm II. agreed to establish the Pépinère, an elite military academy for the rearing of medical personnel. As I will show next, the Pépinère featured prominently in Reil's plans to reform medical education. However, the academy was established clearly in the spirit of the Enlightenment and its teaching faculty was the same as that of the *Collegium medico-chirurgicum*. As Tuchman notes, "There was no idea of *Wissenschaft* and freedom to learn here" (Tuchman 2000: 64). The express aim was to educate medico-surgeons to serve in the Prussian army. Students could study at the academy free of charge and even receive a small stipend if they afterwards committed to serving in the military for eight years.[40] Education at the Pépinière was far more encompassing than at universities of the time. "Its curriculum combined instruction in medicine and surgery, courses in science and basic medical subjects, clinical teaching in the amphitheater, and bedside learning at the Charité" (Bonner 1995: 124). Students of military surgery and medicine had a far greater access to practical training than any university student of medicine could dream of (Hess 2010a: 63). But through its status and the influence of its faculty, the institution represented an idea of academic medicine that opposed any ideals of freedom to teach and learn or the idea to pursue science for its own sake, as the Romantics envisioned it. Reil made use of the academy's practical orientation to argue for the conceptual and institutional separation between medicine as a practical profession and an academic *Wissenschaft*.

The Charité, established in 1727 as a general hospital and teaching clinic, was also dominated by the practical interests of the Prussian state and the King's army. Until well into the first half of the nineteenth century, the hospital remained more or less exclusively for clinical training of students from the military academy. Clinical training as such was a relatively new concept. It dates back only to the second half of the eighteenth century, when the Dutch physician and professor of medicine Herman Boerhaave invented the idea as a form of instruction to practical medicine (Broman 1996: 59–66). By the start of the nineteenth century, the model of the teaching clinic had spread throughout many countries in Europe and began informing important medical centers, such as Berlin or Würzburg. The general idea was to provide medical students with an understanding of their future trade through practical demonstrations on real-life patients (Bonner 1995a: 103–141). Practical instruction existed mainly in the form of apprenticeship prior to the introduction of clinical training. Our knowledge of the history of university clinics remains sketchy (Bleker 1995, Hess 2010a), but there were different modes in which beginning physicians

---

40 Notable alumni, who later moved on to academic science and medicine, include pathologist Rudolf Virchow and physiologist Hermann von Helmholtz.

could receive their practical training: outpatient and polyclinics, where patients were visited and treated in their homes, as well as stationary clinics (Bleker 1995: 91). University clinics would begin to settle on the latter model. As already mentioned, this did not necessarily mean that university students acquired practical hands-on training. University students were graduated to treat patients with virtually no clinical experience. The academic discipline compensated for this lack by redefining the foundations of medical practice, as I will show further down.

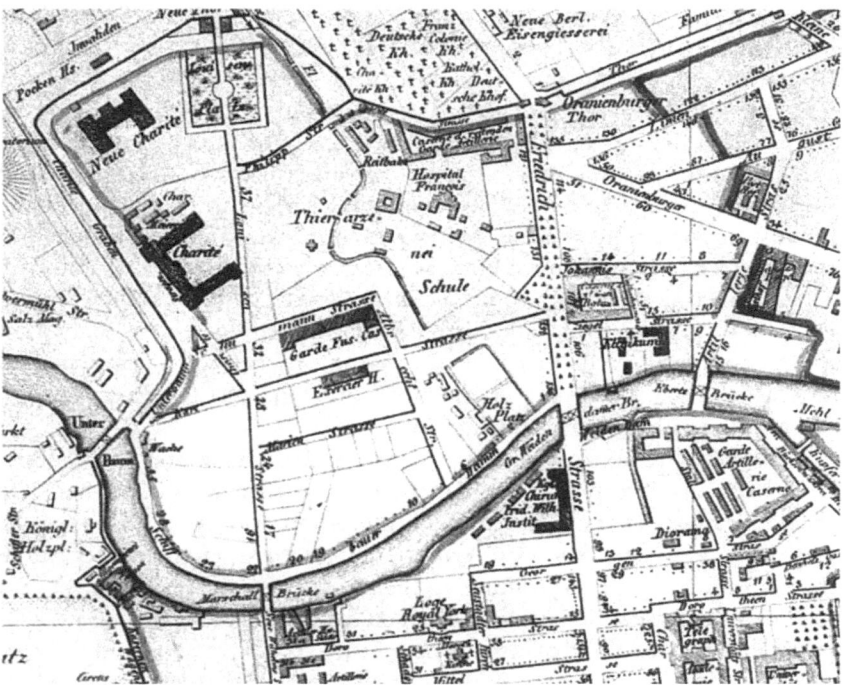

Figure 3.2: *Detail map of Berlin (c. 1839), with the Charité hospital in the upper left corner, the university teaching clinic, center right, on the north banks of the Spree River ("Klinikum"), the Pépinière (aka. Royal Surgical Friedrich-Wilhelm's-Institute) on Friedrichstraße, south of the river, as well as part of the university in the lower right corner. (Source: Volker Hess. 2010. Die Alte Charité, die moderne Irrenabteilung und die Klinik (1790–1820). Die Charité. Geschichte(n) eines Krankenhauses. Ed. Johanna Bleker, Volker Hess. Berlin: Akademie Verlag. p. 65).*

All clinical instruction for students of military medicine and surgery took place at the Charité. And with the establishment of the Pépinière in 1795, the Charité's role as a military teaching clinic was formally cemented (Hess 2010a: 63). The medical faculty of Berlin's new university tried repeatedly to establish strong ties with the Charité hospital for clinical education of their civilian students (Tuchman 2000: 42ff.). But neither King, ministers nor the "shadow medical faculty" would allow university professors of medicine to move their teaching clinics to the hospital. As a result, in 1813, the university faculty founded their own teaching clinic in a building on Ziegelstraße, on the north banks of the Spree River in Berlin (figure 3.2.). Here, Reil established a small "clinical-chemical laboratory", indicating that he wanted to use the clinic also for "higher scientific ends" (Bleker 1995: 96). Even when it was later in the century granted to university faculty to move their teaching clinics to the Charité, students of the military medical academy were still privileged over civilian students (Hess 2010a: 64ff.). However, clinics were still designed purely for instruction at the time. It would take until well into the first half of the nineteenth century until clinical research would become established. Then, the clinical setting would allow professors to study disease empirically and comparatively and thereby contributed to a new theoretical understanding of medicine, next to relaying the ideas of routine medical practice to their students (i.e., diagnosis, working out therapies, making prescriptions, observation and aftercare).

The official reasons given for rejecting inclusion of university clinics into the Charité hospital were that the medical treatment of soldiers had absolute priority over civilian medical care. Another reason was that graduates of the Pépinière were furthermore obliged to an eight-year service in the Prussian army upon completing their studies – this was a clear benefit for the state. Academic physicians looked for employment in larger towns or cities and therefore often moved outside the state where they were educated (Lindeman 1996). A third argument was that military medico-surgeons had to be prepared to treat many wounded soldiers at the same time (Tuchman 2000: 45). In other words, the hospital provided the ideal grounds for equipping students for "mass medicine" (Tuchman 2000: 44); not so much, though, for physicians who were looking to treat bourgeoise and upper-class clients.

In the eighteenth century (and before), most physicians took care merely of an elite of better-off patrons in the urban areas, while most medical practice of the licensed sort fell to surgeons of different ranks, who also treated many of the acute cases (Huerkamp 1985: 44f.).[41] In a still traditionalist vein, learned academic physicians needed to acquire the necessary "*Savoir faire*" for a successful practice, i.e., the bourgeoise manners, the necessary tact and the rhetorical skills to defend a medical standpoint and intervention against a client and his kin (Hess 2010a: 66f.). Next to individual instruction, only a small stationary clinic with a few patients, like a separate ward in the hospital, could provide the appropriate context to learn these qualities, academic physicians believed. This difference in treatment of students and teachers attests to the strong intellectual and institutional divide that existed between the idea of medicine as a learned profession with academic qualities and as a practical profession, which's aim it was to serve the state. A central question therefore is how the new concept of medicine as *Wissenschaft* was able to provide a ground that could harbor elements of both conceptions.

Reil criticized that the state did not have any real plans of how to proceed with the "great masses" (*großer Haufen*) that required medical attention. He lamented that this large bulk of the population was treated mostly by unskilled and only half-qualified practitioners, since they were never brought into contact with medical science in any way or form. However, he did not want to make learned physicians responsible for treating average citizens either (Reil 1804: 12). Instead, his plans revolved around making science or *Wissenschaft* the guiding principle for all of medicine. His ideas for the encompassing reorganization of the medical system thought it unnecessary to distinguish between military and civilian practitioners, and even between medicine and surgery (Reil 1804, 1910). Instead, the only distinction that mattered to him was that between individuals in possession of true science and those merely capable of executing protocols developed on a scientific basis. In the next section I want to highlight the general outlines of Reil's argument.

III. Johann Christian Reil's Plan for Reforming Academic Medicine

Reil developed his plans for reforming academic medicine in Berlin in two pieces of writing: the controversial book with the bulky title *Pepinieren zum Unterricht ärztlicher Routiniers als Bedürfnisse des Staats nach seiner Lage*

---

41 Although non-licensed practitioners were most likely responsible for the bulk of health care of the lower realms of society in eighteenth- and nineteenth-century Germany (Huerkamp 1985: 36ff.).

wie sie ist, published in 1804, and in a memorandum on medical education he wrote in 1807. The latter was later forwarded to Humboldt for his plans to establish the new Berlin university. Humboldt references Reil's ideas in the exposé "On the Organization of the Medical System", written in 1809, which serves as an important document for the founding of the University of Berlin (Humboldt 1964). Reil appears to be performing a form of professional politics in the *Pepinieren*-book, intent on defending the traditional image of the physician as a person of high prestige and privileged to serve only a select few. Accordingly, he grounded his plans for reformation on the contentious assertion that "the learned physician and the wealthy citizen attract each other like amicable poles" (Reil 1804: 9). However, behind these traditionalist-seeming professional intentions lied the far-reaching reorganization of the medical system, which aimed at the institutional separation of the theoretical and practical work of medicine. Guided by the concept of *Wissenschaft*, Reil formulated his plans in the spirit of *Naturphilosophie*, a philosophical current of the Romantic era, spearheaded by Friedrich Wilhelm Joseph Schelling, which sought to place "man" in a universal system of nature.

Schelling's *Naturphilosophie* was decidedly anti-utilitarian and based on the idea of a holistic experience of nature. It combined several elements that made it fitting to argue for the primacy of science over all medical matters. Firstly, the philosophy was abstract enough to keep medical practice at a distance. Broman observes a "comparative absence of narrowly professional concerns in *Naturphilosophie*", although actors "wrote a good deal about health and illness as part of their more general treatments of nature" (Broman 1996: 99). Secondly, despite its transcendental rhetoric, the current was generally open to empirical investigations in a way that would become important for laboratory experiments. For protagonists of *Naturphilosophie*, the structures of reason were essentially equivalent to the structures of nature, and they argued that, with the help of philosophical reason, the science of medicine could bring "an external formal unity to the given and existing manifoldness" of experiences of organic nature (Schelling 1974: 130, see also Broman 1996: 92–96, Zammito 2018: 302–317). The term "organism" reappears in Schelling's and Reil's writings, for example, to simultaneously illustrate the wholeness of the scientific researcher's object of inquiry, namely, nature, but also to signal his own inclusion and participation in the being of nature. In other words, a truly enlightened Romantic natural philosopher could experience (and ultimately understand) nature in himself and through his connection with everything else in the world. *Naturphilosophie* was thus open to insights from empirical sciences, as long as they were organized in a "systematic unity" that was "*prior* in the transcendental sense" (Zammito 2018: 303).[42] As Lynn Nyhart writes about the *Naturphilosoph* Karl Friedrich Burdach: "Only an *Erfahrungswissenschaft* allows us to discover the ways in which the laws of the interior world are played out in the external world and to recognize the inner unity among the diverse particulars of the external world" (Nyhart 1995: 41).

Thirdly, moreover, *Naturphilosophie* incorporated a hierarchy among the sciences, which placed medicine at the top, above all other sciences. The argument was that true scientific physicians experienced the workings of the "God of nature" more closely and directly than any other of the natural sciences could provide (Schelling 1805: v). From 1805 until 1808 Schelling edited the short-lived *Jahrbücher der Medicin als Wissenschaft* together with the physician Adalbert Friedrich Marcus, which gave the program of the Romantic medical reformers its name. In the preface to the first volume, Schelling calls medicine the "crown and bloom of all the natural sciences [*Naturwissenschaften*]" and propagates that

> "philosophers and natural researchers [*Naturforscher*] of all sorts, the chemist and anatomist [*Zergliederer*], the zoologist and physician [*Heilkünstler*], [be] united in a common work, the science [*Wissenschaft*] of the organism, and thereby elevate medicine [*Heilkunde*] to the pinnacle that it should occupy, and gradually advance it" (1805: vi, see also Zammito 2018: 336f.).

As *Wissenschaft*, medicine was thus defined as the queen of all the sciences of nature, from which the various physiological subcurrents and other biological specialties could and would spawn. Likewise, the science itself was composed of various previously existing scientific subdisciplines, which are now directed toward the discipline of medicine. This also shows how the institutional structure of the new university was still confusing. In medicine, professors had previously taught in all the mentioned areas (chemistry, anatomy, zoology), and pursued research individually only in some. Schelling's natural philosophers and the Romantic physicians that followed in his wake were referring to an idea of medicine as a unified science of organic nature and used the category of *Wissenschaft* like many

---

42 In the preface to the *Jahrbuch der Medicin als Wissenschaft*, Schelling argues for the right balance between an "abundance of classical erudition" and a "true experience based on [a] perception of nature [*Naturanschauung*]" (Schelling 1805: xvii).

others of the learned estate to defend a broad enterprise aimed at preserving the intellectual institutions of academic research and teaching (Phillips 2012).

Finally, Schelling's *Naturphilosophie* introduced the crucial distinction between those that (can) possess a true idea of science and experience of nature, and therefore can act autonomously, and those that merely perform tasks delegated to them by some higher authority. In the preface to the *Jahrbücher*, he argues that "he who lacks a thorough perception of nature [*Naturanschauung*] and to whom medicine [*Heilkunde*] has never appeared in relation to general natural research [*allgemeine Naturforschung*]" can hardly be deemed "a learned, or even experienced, physician", now that people have begun to regard the human organism as the "center of nature and the epitome of all its forces"; instead, such individuals can only be "dull *routiniers*", who have internalized the "empty formalism of a theory [...] and thereby the experience of past physicians" (Schelling 1805: xviii).

In Reil's book on *Pepinieren*, the distinction between *routiniers* and true physicians constitutes one of the fundamental differentiations to argue for the establishment of the medical system on the Romantic idea of the natural sciences. He proposed that medical care of the larger part of the population ought to be the responsibility of an estate of medical auxiliaries that he dubbed *routiniers*. These auxiliaries could act both medically and surgically, were useful in both the military and the civilian world and possessed technical skill and mostly only a practicable knowledge of medical science (Heller 1975). Accordingly, the *routinier* "should be able to recognize diseases by their symptoms without really understanding them and to use appropriate medicine without deeper knowledge of their functions" (ibid: 326, see also Broman 1996: 120). These practitioners were effectively molded after the current caste of medico-surgeons, embodying the Enlightenment ideal of medicine as a practical science. And it was suggested that, eventually, "they would replace the practical surgeons, barber surgeons, and apothecaries who failed to meet the health needs of the Prussian people" (Bonner 1995: 24).

Reil's plans argued on two fronts: the pure science basis of medicine and the proper practical education, which would be based on scientific principles. In his book, he made clear demands towards the Prussian state, asking the rhetorical question: "The state sees itself obligated to maintain *academies*, on which *learned* physicians are educated for [treating] rich citizens. Would it then be an unreasonable demand that it also arranges for *Pepinieren*, at which *routiniers* are trained for service of the great masses

[*großen Haufen*]" (Reil 1804: 19)?[43] Admittedly, Reil's plans for two separate and differently oriented medical schools never saw it to fruition. But
his ideas did prefigure the two-tier system of medical research and clinical
care, characteristic of academic medicine today. Humboldt would make a
similar recommendation to Reil's in his 1809 memorandum, speaking of
the complementarity of academic medical institutions and practical training institutions: "Medical agencies [*MedicinalBehörden*] almost inevitably
take a more practical [direction], appropriate for the local circumstances
of their situation, and not a purely scientific [*rein wissenschaftliche*] one;
the faculty-scholars [*FacultaetsGelehrten*] constitute the opposite case. Both
together thus function immensely beneficial [*heilsam*]" (Humboldt 1964:
61).

However, Humboldt structured the medical education system in a three-
fold distinction, which better matches the institutions that developed. He
speaks first of universities as providing "theoretical-scientific [*theoretisch-
wissenschaftlichen*] instruction in relation to the whole area of science [*Wissenschaft*], and with so much practical instruction as is necessary for the
transition from theory to practice and for connection of the two"; second,
of "medical-practical institutions" (*medicinisch-practische Anstalten*) for after
completion of university studies (these included the teaching clinics that
were established in both the Charité and in the university clinic); and third
of "special medical training-schools" (*medicinische SpecialSchulen*), which
include institutions like the current *Pépinière* in Berlin (Humboldt 1964:
62).

What characterized the medical system in Berlin subsequently, as Volker Hess argues, was a double structure, which, "on the one side, had
the clinics of the Charité in a military medicine tradition, and on the
other, the university clinics, which were erected in, and surrounding,
the Ziegelstraße" (Hess 2010a: 68). Nevertheless, I want to show that the
concepts underlying Reil's ideas predetermine our modern understanding
of academic medicine and of medical science. It was not the actual schools
that he envisioned, as we will see, but how he related the different key
actors and the tasks he equipped them with. Hoovering above it all, of

---

43 Literally, Reil speaks of making medical theory as part of the natural sciences
the domain of the academies, which were until the nineteenth century the places
for purely scientific concerns. But as has been shown, Stichweh argues that the
academies experienced an exodus of science at the time, making the universities
the actual places of scientific work (Stichweh 1984: 67ff.). In the onomasiological
perspective, Reil was therefore using an old term for a new thing.

course, was the idea of medicine as a pure science. The rays of *Wissenschaft* came together in the figure of the learned physician, who was a teacher of science and a furtherer of scientific knowledge. Medical care laid mostly in the hands of medical auxiliaries or *routiniers*, who, although themselves separate from pure science, nevertheless attended scientifically founded educational institutions to acquire a proficiency for practice.

IV. A Modern Division of Medical Labor

The distinction between the figure of the *routinier* and that of the learned or scientific physician forms the basis for relating the medical institutions of theory and practice to each other in a uniquely modern fashion. Underlying Reil's (and Humboldt's) plans was the idea that academic physicians could have a medical identity even if they did not participate in treating patients. The bottom line was to frame their tasks in a way that it sustained the scientific practice of medicine and simultaneously contributed to the production of medical practitioners, which could then treat the bulk of the population. Accordingly, *routiniers* were envisioned to serve as auxiliaries to the university-reared physicians. The distribution of tasks between physicians and *routiniers* was based on the notion that the "art of medicine" consisted of two parts "knowledge and action" and that the "transfer [*Mittheilung*] of the art via instruction can only happen in a *double* fashion" (Reil 1804: 20). Either both knowledge and action are taught in its unity (as with learned physicians) or "only the mechanisms of action" themselves (as in the case of the *routiniers*), "without the reasons from which they spring" (Reil 1804: 20). All other distinctions, for instance, those between military and civilian, or medical and surgical schools, Reil condemned as either "unessential [*außerwesentlich*]" or even "senseless" (ibid.).

Consequently, for Reil, the *routinier* was characterized "partly by *the mechanism of action*, [and] partly by *his restriction to the respective sphere in which he is to serve as a tool*" (Reil 1804: 62). He calls them "psychological automata" that are aware of the rules according to which they act, but that are "without awareness [*Bewußtsein*]" of the "construction of the same from their [scientific] principles" (Reil 1804: 63). Though the phrasing of both Reil and Schelling would suggest a derogative understanding of these medical auxiliaries, both were in fact elevating them above all existing medical practitioners of the time – except university physicians. Reil even admits that it is difficult to draw a "clear boundary [*scharfe Gränze*] between him [i.e., the *routinier*] and the scientific physician" (Reil 1804: 62). The reason is that both are exposed in their own way to medicine as science, something that most of current practitioners lacked in the eyes of the reformers. If we were to map Reil's distinction onto current circumstances, the roles of *routiniers* are conceptually precursory to those of today's clinicians and physicians in private practice. These practitioners treat much of the population and practice based on scientific principles, but they do not themselves contribute actively to advancing the science of medicine. Reil's academic physicians, in turn, would today resemble medical scientists holding MDs (or PhDs, respectively) and devoted entirely to research. It was this distinction – between those that actively furthered the science of medicine and those that merely acted on the scientific basis established thereby – that was at the heart of Reil's reform ideas, rather than any concrete roles or institutions he described.

The relative proximity that Reil constructed between the physician and the *routinier* had implications for the organization of the medical system. He strictly opposed the idea that all medical practitioners should become learned physicians. In fact, a horde of academic physicians would not be favorably equipped to serve the bulk of the population in his opinion. In a revealing passage, he argues that too much "rationalism" hampers proper praxis and that "the tactful routinier, whom nature has given practical genius, so often acts far better than the superfine theoretician" (Reil 1804: 24, see also 93). Through this classification, he even grants *routiniers* qualities that were formerly restricted to practicing physicians. Reil admits to them the status of being better practitioners (at least when it comes to treating the large part of the population, as the state required it; but it would seem also for medical practice as such). While learned physicians were too caught up with their medical theories and rhetorical eloquence, the medical auxiliaries would instead recognize disease when they saw it and know how to act immediately. These practitioners should therefore have their proper place next to the academic physician, he demanded (ibid.).

By elevating the practical qualities of the *routinier* above those of the learned physician, Reil was simultaneously making an argument for a division of labor within the medical system. Although it was granted that both university doctors and *routiniers* could actively function as healers (within their respective purviews), the true task of the physician, according to Reil, was nevertheless defined as pursuing *Wissenschaft* – without any regard for its practical potential or utilizing it for external ends. This also reflected in his ideas for the organization of medical education: "The learned physician must go to a *university*, which teaches science

[*Wissenschaft*] in its organic unity, whereas the routinier must be reared in a *Pepiniere*, which organizes the raw material according to its future purpose and teaches the mechanisms of action [*Mechanismus des Handelns*] solely for external purposes" (Reil 1804: 28). However, Reil implied that it would be the same faculty teaching future learned physicians and medical auxiliaries. This implication made any factual distinction between medical academy (*qua* university) and practical training school – to use Reil's word – unessential.[44]

A teacher at a training school had to be a "philosopher and scientific physician", in order to be able to construct the subject of his teachings "in its entirety [*Ganzen*] and from the whole [*Ganzen*]" (Reil 1804: 93). This is a clear affirmation of *Naturphilosophie* ideals and of *Wissenschaft* as a holistic natural experience. Reil claimed that not the material taught, but the manner of education, distinguished between "true" medical students *qua* scientists and medical auxiliaries. "Whereas the presentation to medical students should be 'learned' and 'critical,' *Routiniers* should be taught in a manner that is 'popular' and 'dogmatic'" (Broman 1989: 45, s. Reil 1804: 94). The boundary that Reil drew was supposed to correspond to the intellectual quality of the student and represented an idea of Romantic elitism that distinguished the free-thinking scientific "genius", who could immerse himself (ingeniousness of this sort was also seen as restricted to the male population in the early nineteenth century) in *Wissenschaft*, from the confined mind that listened only to doctrine and accordingly was uncreative (Schaffer 1990, see also Tuchman 1993: 27f.).

This ideology subsequently became institutionalized in medical education in concrete terms. The first prominent generation of medical scientists like Johannes Müller,[45] manifested a practice in which they hand-picked individuals from the pool of medical students and offered them extracurricular training in medical research if they saw them fit for forming the future elite cadre of scientists (Coleman 1988: 39, see also Lenoir 1997:

---

44 Although in a very short paragraph he states that "The Pepiniere should not be at the same place as a university, so that the conceit [*Dünkel*] of the academic does not awaken the envy [*Scheelsucht*] of the routinier and tempt him to defect" (Reil 1804: 89).

45 Müller is best remembered as a rigorous experimental researcher, who trained a cadre of people in his Berlin laboratory in the 1830s and 1840s that would become eminent figures in nineteenth-century science and medicine – including Emil du Bois-Reymond, Hermann von Helmholtz, Jacob Henle, Theodor Schwann and Rudolf Virchow (Otis 2007). He will play a role again briefly in the next chapter.

103f.). But there is no need for further concern with the underlying philosophy, which had Reil convinced that the *routinier* "possesses *Wissenschaft* merely as an artifice and *in concreto*", as opposed to the physician (Reil 1804: 64, see also Broman 1989: 45). What is central, though, is the idea that the two groups would receive and acquire different things from the *same* faculty and courses. Despite Reil's insistence on differentiation, all students, at least initially, had to be taught as equals. An education in *Wissenschaft* was thereby regarded as propaedeutic no matter if students would become practitioners or scientists. Refracted onto the circumstances of today, we can say that the plans of reformers like Reil prevailed not in the factual institutions that were erected in its aftermath, but in the inner logic of how they saw science, practice and teaching relate.

V. The New Physiology as Modern Medicine's Scientific Culture

How could *Wissenschaft* be taught at the turn of the nineteenth century? How did it act propaedeutically for medical students? And how were existing medical institutions reformed in the process? What was the scientific culture that henceforth determined the actions of learned physicians *qua* medical scientists? Reil and the Romantic reformers were still looking for answers to these questions prior to the founding of the University of Berlin. In his memorandum to Humboldt, he was lamenting the current state of medical education in Germany, described above. He wrote:

> "*Medicine* is [the] natural science [*Naturkunde*] of organisms in their interrelations to the environment, applied to the end of healing their diseases. – Natural science is its *basis*, application its *specific nature*. [...] At no university is [the] natural science [*Naturkunde*] of organisms taught as a *pure science* [*Wissenschaft*]: systematically self-contained, removed from everything alien, and as an end in itself. It is always only taught as *medicine*, i.e., as an applied science [*Scienz*] towards the particular end of healing; thus, only those parts [are taught,] which are suitable for application – and these in a disgustingly meticulous detail and interspersed with rules that refer to the art [*Technik*]" (Reil 1910: 52).[46]

He complained that medical education focused too narrowly on teaching those parts that are "suitable for application" or which refer only to the

---

46 Unless otherwise noted, all translations from the German are my own.

"art" or "technique".[47] This neglected the crucial aspect of expanding the pure science or *Wissenschaft* of medicine. "Either one thus has to", he suggested, "restrict medicine entirely to the art [*Technik*] (where it then loses its place within the organism of the sciences [*Wissenschaften*]) or to unite it with the subject of natural knowledge [*Naturerkenntnisse*]" (ibid: 53). As a scientific subject, in other words, medicine had to establish itself as a general and encompassing scientific discipline. It needed to be treated by practitioners as an end in itself, devoted solely to "cultivating the sciences [*Wissenschaften*]", and not simply as a sideshow like it was for most professors (Reil 1910: 50, 58). It was common for them to be teachers of medicine at a university next to their practice. "This science [*Scienz*], which propounds the principles of the natural doctrine [*Naturlehre*] of all organisms as such, is the indispensable propaedeutic of every particular [science], therefore also of the natural doctrine [*Naturlehre*] of human nature" (ibid: 60).

What the rhetoric of the pure science ideal associated with the Prussian reformers admittedly tends to obscure, is that, though its proponents sought to liberate themselves from issues of practical relevance, it did not mean they abandon the relationship to practice altogether. To conform to the beliefs of their day, they rather reinvented the relationship by reversing the hierarchy that the Enlightenment had set up, so that activities in pure science became the precondition for practical life. What was essential in this regard, was that, as Phillips notes, the new category of *Wissenschaft* "contained folded within itself the essence of all practical knowledge" (2012: 105, see also Kaldewey 2013: 294–306). Seeing how medical physiologists began treating problems independently from clinical concerns, social historians of nineteenth-century German medicine and science regard that the identity of medical science turned into a biological one, separating it from the institution of medical practice. Rather than seeing how the emergence of the term *Wissenschaft* indicated the detachment of pure science inquiries from medicine, the question is how the subject allowed them to maintain their role as medical teachers.

The general organization of disciplines in the newly emerging university landscape followed the pure science ideal, the pursuit of scientific questions in freedom and unhampered by the expectation of practical outcomes. Stichweh shows that this included a reversal of the hierarchy between the philosophical faculty as a propaedeutic teaching institution

---

47 For the difficulties of rendering the German word 'Technik' in the late-eighteenth century into English see Schatzberg (2018: 11ff., 102f.).

and the traditional faculties of law, medicine and theology, which trained learned professionals (Stichweh 1984: 31ff.). This moved humanities fields like history, philology and philosophy to the top of the hierarchy, while the disciplines of the natural sciences began distinguishing between their pure and practical parts to secure a position in the disciplinary hierarchy. While disciplines in the philosophical faculty like chemistry or physics had often served as auxiliary sciences to the higher faculties, they now constituted their own autonomous disciplines with a research imperative. Stichweh argues that this reversal reflected in a new orientation of the disciplines to each other: The philosophical faculty became autonomous and, under the banner of *Wissenschaft*, the new locus for scientific research, giving birth to the modern system of academic disciplines. At the same time, the faculties of law, medicine and theology began to orient themselves towards "problems of professional practice and education" (Stichweh 1984: 36). As I have been arguing, however, the formerly higher faculties also need to be regarded – at least in the case of medicine – as becoming places of pure science. Rather than constituting a neat distinction between *Wissenschaft* and professional praxis, medicine began to form a scientific discipline that combined the interests of both. I will mention in the next chapter how one strategy to argue for the academic autonomy of the medical discipline was to borrow features from the natural sciences like physics or chemistry, which were now housed in the philosophical faculty.

None of the fields that developed after the turn of the nineteenth century had the clear distinctions that we know of academic disciplines today. And only few had their departments and granted disciplinary degrees. For instance, virtually all research in medical fields and in areas of organic biology was conducted by individuals holding doctoral degrees in medicine. As mentioned already above, as long as actors remained part of the medical faculty, they also remained academic teachers of medicine, even if their research interests shifted to problems that prepared those of the morphological zoologists. In the old academic system of early Modernity, what distinguished academic physicians professionally was their "license to both teach *and* practice medicine" (Broman 1996: 52, see also Broman 1989: 60). As teachers, they lectured to students on the theoretical doctrines of the medical tradition. Professors tried to move up from the lower philosophical faculty into a higher faculty and, within the medical faculty, through virtually the entire canon of medical topics in correspondence to seniority (from "practical" subjects like pharmacology or surgery through botany and chemistry up to the theoretical fields of anatomy, pathology and physiology). Now, at the start of the nineteenth century, in contrast, this system was abolished for one in which they remained within a fixed subject orbit throughout their career (ibid: 177, see also Nyhart 1995: 53f., Stichweh 1984: 33). As a result, the professors who devoted themselves to the science of organic nature had to find a way to sell their function as medical teachers so that it would also conform with their developed set of specialized research interests.

As the foundational science of medicine, physiology was for many interested in pure science research the area of choice. However, physiology was not yet neatly distinguished as a homogenous discipline. Rather, the science comprised a row of different approaches and questions, ranging from human anatomy and pathology all the way to zoology. There were many different attempts to homogenize the discipline at the time. But it seems that the current of *Naturphilosophie* acted best to unify the natural sciences generally (Phillips 2012: Schauz 2020: 152ff.), and physiology especially (Zammito 2018: 318ff.). From tradition, physiology was ranked a primary academic subject of medicine because it had the highest philosophical appeal and laid the theoretical foundation for all the other medical subjects. Therefore, it was not (yet) a special method or set of fundamental questions that defined physiology. It was rather the idea of a holistic understanding of the true nature of organic life, which it was believed could be experienced through the study of natural *qua* physiological phenomena. In the first generation of medical researchers, many therefore held joint chairs and taught in different areas, which complemented and overlapped each other. Johannes Müller, for example, held the chair in physiology and comparative anatomy at the University of Berlin from 1833 onward. He taught students in anatomy, pathology and physiology, while publishing research in all three areas as well as in zoology and even marine biology.[48] This goes to show how ill-defined physiology was as a discipline at the start of the nineteenth century. Only in the second half of the nineteenth century did physiology begin to be properly institutionalized (Kramer 2009). When looking at physiology in the following, it needs to accordingly be kept in mind that it is the name for a collective field of medical sciences. What characterized the role of the new professors of medicine as teachers subsequently was especially the practical engagement with the science of physiology (in whatever concrete fashion or form).

The elevation of medicine to a pure science discipline, separate from all immediate practical concerns, thus became enshrined in a new un-

---

48 Nonetheless, he regarded himself primarily as an anatomist and is conventionally categorized as one (Otis 2007).

derstanding of the science of physiology, which acted as the unifying center of what Schelling called the "natural science of organisms". To understand how the new professors maintained their relationship to practical medicine, requires drawing on the concept of disciplines, particularly in their socializing function. As I argued in the previous chapter, disciplines can be understood not only as communities centred around an epistemic object, but rather also as communities defined by a shared scientific culture and professional *habitus*. They combine the function of research and teaching – a concept introduced with the new ideology of *Wissenschaft* – which can be refined to mean the integration of scientific contemplation and practical education in a given scientific culture. Disciplines furthermore orient themselves towards certain societal or cultural demands, which they do by adhering to specific conceptual categorizations like "pure and applied science" or "science and art". The question then is how the laboratory science of physiology was able to provide a culture for the discipline of medicine that could satisfy both the outlook to medical practice and to scientific research.

One angle of how this was possible, was in the transformation of the concept of practice (table 3.3). The idea of practice that defined the learned physician changed on the side of medical science – turning the professor's praxis from the practice of medicine into the practice of physiological research. While physiology thus became cognitively independent in terms of research, it was also framed as a form of practical engagement (and no longer as a set of theoretical doctrines) that could at the same time prepare the prospective practitioner and provide the basis for *Bildung*, the cultural (self-)formation of the student's character destined to devote a life to *Wissenschaft* (Coleman 1988, s. also Kremer 2009: 354). It is no coincidence, then, that by the 1820s many medical faculties in Germany were teaching physiology as an experimental science (Bonner 1995a: 154f.).

This new understanding of physiology can be traced to its origins in the *Archiv für Physiologie*, which Reil launched in 1795. The periodical is significant because it was the first European journal devoted to the specialty. Reil employed the *Archiv* to lay the theoretical foundations for a unifying science of medicine in the understanding of *Wissenschaft* and addressed a more or less clearly defined scientific community (Broman 1991, see also 1989: 39ff., 1996: 86f.). It can be disregarded here that the periodical was started first in a Kantian vein and that its protagonist only later adopted the stance of *Naturphilosophie* (ibid: 22f.). From my vantage point, it can nonetheless show how medicine changed from resting on physiological doctrines to being based on a complex scientific culture, which gave medical students practical and cognitive qualities through experimental engagement with organic nature. For this purpose, I want to sketch how physiology, in relation to anatomy, transitioned into being an experimental science.

	learned and rational medicine		craft medicine
Traditional medicine	teaching (doctrines)	practice (internal medicine)	surgery
Enlightenment medicine	practical sciences ——> medico-surgery		
Medicine as Wissenschaft	teaching (scientific culture)	practice (pure science)	internal medicine, surgery
	medical science		**clinical practice**

Table 3.3: Changes in theoretical and practical occupations of modern medicine prior to the nineteenth century (my depiction).

According to historian of medicine Andrew Cunningham, who has uncovered what he calls the disciplinary identities of "old" physiology and anatomy in a pair of papers entitled "The pen and the sword", the relationship between both until the end of the eighteenth century was that of a theoretical science and a practical art. This division of intellectual labor corresponded to the premodern conviction that mental work was noble and of high esteem, while manual work, in contrast, pointed to its practitioners lowly and humble status (Cunningham 2002: 635). Physiology, as the theory about the causes of living things, relied on the visual evidence provided by anatomy. Conceptually, it was not subjected to anatomical discoveries, but only to the general changes and fashions of the dominating natural philosophies (ibid: 641). Thus, while anatomy comprised the art of dissecting, physiological contemplation itself did not include such activities. Physiology was neither investigative, "nor an empirical discipline, nor an experimental discipline. It was, by contrast, a thinking and talking discipline – a discourse" (ibid: 645). Anatomy, in turn, constituted an investigative and experimental discipline, which complemented the physiological discourse with teachings of organic forms and structures (Cunningham 2003: 59f., see also 2002: 648). Its aim was to investigate and classify the parts of the body and it thereby could only suggest to physiology the viability of theoretical conclusions about an organism's vital functions (Cunningham 2002: 658). The crucial point for Cunningham is that, while physiology depended on anatomical experiments, it was itself not an experimental discipline before the nineteenth century.

However, by the eighteenth century, the premodern prejudices about the contrasting moral status of physiology and anatomy largely dissipated, as physiological work became evermore dependent on anatomical dissections and experiments. A famous example is the Swiss scholar Albrecht von Haller. For Zammito, Haller represented the indivisible unity of anatomical doctrines of organic structure and of physiological teachings of animation and he therefore constituted a crucial moment on the path toward the modern life sciences (2018: 79–91). Haller indeed had a reputation as an industrious and sophisticated experimenter. "The sheer quantity of animal experimentation that Haller undertook, and his dedication to experiment as his 'oracle', would seem to indicate that the experimental physiologist had [with him] at last arrived" (Cunningham 2002: 653). But Haller kept the two professional roles clearly separated and the disciplinary distinction between old anatomy and physiology clearly intact. On the one hand, he was engaged in physiological theorizing in such works as his *First Lines of Physiology*, published in 1751, about the forces inaccessible to the senses that were responsible for enabling organic function and movement (ibid: 654f.). On the other hand, a separate set of interests guided his *Dissertation on the Sensible and Irritable Parts of Animals* (1755), which concerned the anatomical activity of finding new ways to divide and classify the parts of bodies (Cunningham 2003: 66). Moreover, as Cunningham explains, Haller made the distinction between both disciplines explicit himself by placing an engraving depicting the activities of the anatomist and physiologist on the front of the second volume – published in 1760 – of his *Elements of Physiology of the Human Body* (figure 3.4). While the left side shows the "manual *art* of anatomy", the right side depicts "the mental *science* of physiology":

> The anatomist cuts, the physiologist reflects. The anatomist is active, knife in hand. The physiologist writes, in the conventional philosopher's pose with cheek on hand. The anatomist deals with means, the physiologist with ends. The anatomising is about *what* and *how*, the physiologising is about *why*. The anatomist deals in *findings* and *experiments*, while the physiologist deals with *causes*, something not accessible to the anatomist" (Cunningham 2002: 655).

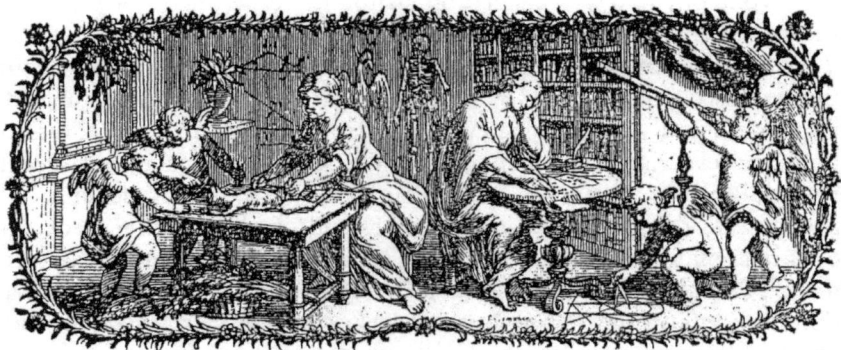

Figure 3.4: Depictions of the activities of anatomy (left) and physiology (right) – frontispiece to volume two of Albrecht von Haller's Elementa Physiologiae
Corporis Humanae (1760). (Source: Andrew Cunningham. 2002. The
pen and the sword: Recovering the disciplinary identity of physiology and
anatomy before 1800 I: Old physiology – the pen. Studies in History and
Philosophy of the Biological and Biomedical Sciences 33, p. 655).

For Haller, therefore, the physiologist of his time presupposed qualities
of an anatomist since he theoretically deduced function from the sensible
evidence of anatomical experiment. But philosophical ideas of function
were not themselves induced through experiment. Since it was, in short,
no longer inappropriate for a thinker to also get his hands dirty, Haller
could engage in both the manual and the discursive activities without violating their boundaries. Irrespective of the historical issue whether Haller
constituted the first experimental physiologist or not, Cunningham shows
how the modern discipline incorporated elements of both old anatomy
and physiology, art and science, or practice and theory, to form "a new and
distinctive discipline, with new goals, standards, procedures, ideology and
products" (Cunningham 2002: 661). His elaborations thus seem to echo
my argument about the reinvention and reintegration into medicine of the
distinctions between theory and practice.

Broman aptly observes that Reil's *Archiv* is the locus in which this
recombination first publicly occurred. Whether or not understood as
such at the outset, the periodical quickly evolved into a program for a
unified *Wissenschaft* of medicine in the style of Schelling's *Naturphilosophie*
(Broman 1991: 30ff., see also Zammito 2018: 283). Through the research
program it cultivated, it reveals how the formerly distinct interests of
function (physiology), and form (anatomy) became expressions of one

and the same transcendental natural process. While previously physiology provided the cause of anatomical form, or form represented the "formal or efficient cause of function"; after 1800, "*Naturphilosophie* provided the theoretical framework for examination of organic form for its own sake, as the external manifestation of physiological process" (ibid: 35). As a result, actors were able to integrate the practice of scientific experimentation into a general activity of theorizing about the form and function of organic nature without breaching disciplinary boundaries.

Accordingly, someone like Ignaz Döllinger, as the last in a long tradition of forbearers to the nineteenth-century science of biology, could now hold the first modern chair for both anatomy and physiology in a German medical faculty – namely, at the University of Würzburg in 1806 – and link the theoretical study of animal form to the microscopic analysis of organic matter (Zammito 2018: 340–352).[49] His chair is thus a model for the one Müller would receive in 1833. For this reason, the *Archiv* is seen to have provided a platform for the rise of morphology, which constituted itself in a "self-conscious disciplinary community" and defended its research program "against the constrains of [medical] practice" (Broman 1996: 188, 1991: 29–36, Zammito 283ff., see also Nyhart 1995: 53ff.). Thus, although Reil initially intended to never lose "contact with the clinical and practice aspects of medicine", his periodical nevertheless evolved into being devoted primarily to a research program for studying animal form (Broman 1991: 22). As Zammito notes, "the *Archiv* proved to be a journal dedicated to the special research program of physiology, apart from medical application" (2018: 285).

For scholars like Broman and Zammito this development thus acts as proof that physiology's identity transitioned from medicine to biology and not that its research culture enabled the establishment of medicine as an independent scientific discipline. The main reason for this assumption is that the medical theory the journal ended up propelling was apparently no longer designed to provide principles for clinical action. Zammito simply claims a general lapse in medicine's interest in *Naturphilosophie* in the first decade of the nineteenth century and a return to empirical grounds for forming clinical guidance (ibid: 339). But Broman thinks more specifically that, in the process of the discipline's transformation, "physiological writing in German Europe began to lose its intimate connection with medical pedagogy" (1991: 35). Given the occupational differentiation in medicine

---

49 As Lynn Nyhart shows, by mid-century efforts were made to again separate the disciplines of anatomy and physiology institutionally (1995: 67–80).

discussed above, he wonders how the medical profession was able to maintain a façade of professional unity at all (Broman 1996: 193). His answer is that as professors of medicine these practitioners of a *new* science also continued to lecture on *old* subjects like anatomy to students studying in the medical faculty – a situation that could not endure, prompting the institutional transition from medicine to biology later in the century (Broman 1991: 38). I want to suggest instead that, while physiology indeed acquired a new identity, this did not mean the loss of its identity as a science of medicine. By interlacing the former distinction between anatomy as an art and physiology as science, the theoretical discourse of physiology was now complemented by specific experimental practices – a scientific culture and *habitus* that medical research practitioners could clearly identify with. Therefore, to transmit this culture to following generations, the general form of medical pedagogy changed from disputations and lectures to the practical engagement of students in the laboratory with the research subject of physiology.

VI. The Function of Medicine as a Modern Academic Discipline

With this reformed sense of physiology as an experimental science, the modern discipline of medicine was now able to accomplish its combined research and teaching functions. Naturally, its medical identity not only implied the role of securing recruitment into the ranks of medical science practitioners; it at the same time meant remaining faithful to the idea of the medical professor as an educator of practicing doctors. However, the medical course was not yet divided into prospective researchers and physicians. In fact, physiological research would only become professionalized towards the end of the century, allowing for its own track of academic education and degree garneting programs (Kremer 2009: 345). In other words, professors were confronted with only a homogenous group of medical students, which acted as the resource for both a small elite of individuals they regarded as qualified to join the ranks of medical science and for the group that would move on to become practicing physicians. To fully understand how the discipline of medicine was able to serve this double requirement, I want to examine more closely the pedagogical ideology behind the ideas of the Romantic medical academics.

The connecting element behind the Romantic pedagogical ideology was the empirical experience of nature, as it was brought by laboratory science. For Reil's auxiliaries *qua* medical practitioners, this science could contribute to "a system of rules, provided for living conception [*Anschauung*], which is formed to an organism on the lower sphere of the real as a regulative to action" (Reil 1804: 64). For those that fit the category of *Wissenschaft*, however, the experience would not only be in demonstration and academic discourse, but also in the self-consciousness of the learned student, in his experience of the wholeness of the transcendental being, which in *Naturphilosophie* was called nature or God. In his book on *Pepinieren*, Reil wrote that the scientific teacher "lets nature, as it were, emerge in front of the eyes of his pupils" (Riel 1804: 33) – both in himself, as an example of nature, but also in his demonstrations. More, the introduction to laboratory practice would also allow those hand-picked students aspiring to become professors themselves to keep the educational demonstrations in class going as well as to pursue their own philosophical questions with the aid of experiment. This form of holistic education was enshrined in the pedagogical concept of *Bildung*, as the formation and education of moral citizens, astute practitioners and truly enlightened minds.

Since the late eighteenth century, the concept of *Bildung* had encouraged the study of Classical – especially Greek – languages and thought as a model for moral and intellectual character development also in the "modern" world (Coleman 1988: 45). In contrast to learnedness, which had characterized embodiment of a higher profession essentially through a solitary and contemplative ideal since the Middle Ages, the category of *Bildung* suggested that a university education would produce graduates more generally directed towards an idea of the common good (Kaldewey 2013: 300). According to Koselleck's historical analysis, the concept simultaneously emerged from the context of the Enlightenment and was a significant reaction against its ideology (2006: 110, 116ff., 327f.). As a child of the Enlightenment, *Bildung* was a category directed at society and public life: "Personal self-formation leads to action-guiding behavior", Koselleck states; "*Bildung* does not lead to contemplative passivity, but compels one to communicative actions, forces the vita activa" (ibid: 119).

Still, the category departed from the Enlightenment's strict pragmatic and vocational idea of university training and propagated the values of not specialized, but of a broad and more general education. "The *Bildung* of rational thinking," Schelling wrote in his *Lectures on the Method of Academic Study*, "by which I mean not merely a superficial getting used to [*Angewöhnung*], but a *Bildung* that passes into the [very] essence of the human being, [...] is also the only [*Bildung*] toward rational acting" (1974: 31). Stated differently, natural researchers and physicians at the start of the century stylized the holistic university education that resulted in *Bildung* as a at the same time the prerequisite for a mentality befitting the practicing doctor *and* as a source of innovation and novelty for the researcher. For physicians, the concept therefore helped secure their academic status, because *Bildung* and learnedness both worked similarly to make a university education the marker of the academic doctor's identity. "Only now", as Broman notes, "that education formed the foundation of physicians' corporate prestige not because of the erudition it conferred, but instead because of the depth of character and quality of insight it developed in the student" (1996: 72, see also Turner 1980: 118). Physiology, as a modern science combining experimental practices and theoretical knowledge, provided the possibility for the *Bildung* of a harmonious and integrated personality in the student, because it required the contemplation of an equally harmonious and integrated object – organic nature (Phillips 2012: 150).

I will wrap up this investigation of medicine's function as an academic discipline with a telling example of how physiology was seen as the appropriate science to offer such an education. For this purpose, historian William Coleman (1988) provides an excellent case study of Jan Evangelista Purkyně at the University of Breslau (today's Wrocław). In 1839, Purkyně created the first physiological institute for medical education in the German lands. But even before that, as Coleman shows, after his arrival in Breslau in 1823, he used physiology to institutionalize the training of aspiring physicians and researchers through practical engagement with organic nature, since it took "man as its principal subject" and represented a "synthesis of all the natural sciences" (Coleman 1988: 27). Coleman's case questions the conventional primacy of the philosophical faculty of the reformed German university and thereby also the change in physiology's identity from medical to biological. His study therefore allows realizing how physiology became reframed as an experimental science out of pedagogical reasons in the wake of restructuring medicine as *Wissenschaft*. This provided medical researchers with a professional mark and a means to install recruitment structures in the medical faculty, which had become itself a hub of pure science after the start of the nineteenth century.

Purkyně was a follower of the late-eighteenth century educational reformer Johann Heinrich Pestalozzi and believed, in contrast to the neo-humanists, "that individual development could, and emphatically should, follow upon close engagement with the natural world and the realia of daily life and should not be confined to or even emphasize the cultural ideals of ancient Greece" (ibid: 30). Textbook learning alone could never be satisfying in bringing the subject of the natural sciences to students. Instead, Purkyně developed a hands-on understanding of training in science and research since he believed that a cultural self-formation could not be sufficiently achieved through textual exegesis alone. His innovation was to move the training of students "from an era of lectures and reading [...] to another world, to the world of the classic scientific institute, in which he who learns, the student, becomes the principal agent of his own instruction" (ibid: 27). As a result, an institute like that in Breslau was able to attend to the requirements of both of the new medical occupations: it provided, on the one hand, a proper education in the natural sciences for students, who would go on to enter medical practice, as most apparently did (ibid: 16). "The self-involvement of the student and the creation of an institutional basis for such involvement", on the other, "opened the way to the possibility that the student might elect to follow a career in medical or scientific research" (ibid: 40, see also Olesko 1988: 313).

In sum, it can be said that the plan to reform the medical system under the category of medicine as *Wissenschaft*, as envisioned by Reil, laid the conceptual and institutional foundation for an academic discipline of medical science. From a research cultural point of view, which was exemplified by the pedagogical ideology of *Bildung*, the discipline functioned to provide different future practitioners with the necessary *habitus* for their individual roles in medicine, whether it was the learned physician or the medical professor, who was also a researcher on fundamental biological issues. The new physiology, as the central field of engagement for practitioners in medical science was able to provide the scientific discipline of medicine with occupational autonomy, while simultaneously securing for it a structural affiliation to the medical faculty at a time when a doctorate in medicine was still a requirement for both practicing physicians and medical scientists.

4. An Applied Science Between Laboratory and Clinic – Scientific Medicine in Mid-Nineteenth-Century Germany

When there is mention of "scientific medicine" in the historical literature, it is mostly used as a generic term describing virtually all forms of (modern) science-based medicine before the age of biomedicine. What is thereby obscured, as I will demonstrate in this chapter and the next, is that the German version – *wissenschaftliche Medicin* – as well as the English rendering each indicated very specific and historically bounded programs. I pointed out in the introduction that especially for English-speaking historians, scientific medicine means a variety of different science-based approaches to medicine, ranging from rationalistic systems of pathology and therapeutics in the eighteenth century through application of natural history to the clinic in the early-nineteenth century to medicine grounded in experimental laboratory science (Hagner 2003, Warner 1995). All these programs did indeed make claims to scientificity, but they did not use the moniker of scientific medicine to make these claims. The Anglo-American renderings of the concept of scientific medicine have led to some confusion in the case of nineteenth-century German science and medicine, on which I focus here.[50] How has that occurred?

The analytical use of the term scientific medicine by scholars to describe the German context actually turns out to be somewhat of a false friend. The English-language use differs considerably from the German meaning. While the Anglo-American understanding of scientific medicine comprised a broad category, the German term for scientific medicine (*wissenschaftliche Medicin*) represents a very specific program, which competed with other contemporaneous programs over the dominant description of academic medicine and medical science around the mid-nineteenth century. But social historians of science and medicine in the Anglo-American tradition understand scientific medicine as a general form of German academic medicine, which developed since mid-century centered on the

---

50 The concept is usually placed into the context of the political and industrial modernization of the German states in the second half of the nineteenth century, in which also the general social and cultural appreciation of natural science is said to have increased (Lenoir 1997: 75–130, Tuchman 1993, see also Hagner 2003: 65ff., Olesko 1988: 323f.).

laboratory and the broadly construed field of experimental physiology (Hagner 2003, Lenoir 1997: 96–130, Tuchman 1993: 54–90). Michael Hagner therefore speaks of a "grand narrative or epic of scientific medicine", which "worked remarkably well in overshadowing the various, sometimes contradictory, meanings of scientific medicine and the sharp conflicts between the bench and the bedside" (Hagner 2003: 85f.). We need to of course consider that Hagner's use of the term scientific medicine here conforms to the analytical understanding in Anglo-American discourses. But what he means is that historians have constructed a (false) coherent image of academic medicine in the second half of the nineteenth century in which practices in the laboratory and the clinic were united by the science of physiology. Next to being a lab science proper, physiology at the time acted as "a model for clinical medicine", lending it "experimental approaches, instruments, and measuring devices", and, even more broadly, as a phenomenon "omnipresent in nineteenth-century discourse and culture" (ibid: 66f.).

The ubiquity of physiology has thus obscured the heterogeneity of the scientific programs for medicine that flourished around the mid-nineteenth century. Historians concerned with German medicine in the nineteenth century acknowledge that the individual programs "differed in their emphasis on key elements" but contend nonetheless that "there was essential agreement on the core of their proposed scientific medicine" (Lenoir 1997: 105, Tuchman 1993: 77, 80). In short, while the science of physiology has dominated historical narratives of science and medicine in the second half of the nineteenth century, for historians the concept of scientific medicine also functions as one of Harris's "supercategories" – integrating the different currents of clinical and laboratory science of the time into a common denominator. This has in no small part complicated the uncovering of medicine's disciplinary identity. Therefore, the task here is to untangle the different competing programs and to trace the conceptual origins of scientific medicine in Germany. This chapter is devoted to discussing the different programs of medical science, which around mid-century constituted a confusing constellation comprising elements like the laboratory, the clinic, competing methodologies, and the sciences of physiology and pathology. What enabled the historical concept of scientific medicine to become the dominant idea of a science-based medicine? And what did it entail if we look behind the grand narratives of experimental physiology?

The programs that were popular around mid-century all relied on physiology in different ways – even the emerging concept of clinical medicine took recourse to practices coming from the new laboratory science. But these programs were nevertheless divided by their conceptions of scientific knowledge production, and therefore also by their understandings of the relationship between science and medical practice, the lab and the clinic. And whereas scientific medicine has become closely associated with the science of physiology in historiographical epics and narratives, as a historical program, as I will demonstrate, the primary science associated with scientific medicine was in fact *not* physiology, but pathology. Prominent programs at the time that relied heavily on the science of physiology were referred to as *rationelle Medicin* (Henle 1844) or *physiologische Heilkunde* (Roser/Wunderlich 1842). These programs – especially that of physiological medicine by Karl Wunderlich and his Tübingen allies, Wilhelm Roser and Wilhelm Griesinger – stressed the measurement of *normal* physiological processes and introduced laboratory-inspired instruments to the clinic. Volker Hess speaks of "proto-statistical methods" through which clinicians, inspired by the physical sciences, would record clinical phenomena like fever over extended periods and try to evaluate them scientifically (2010b: 91). As he states, it was about "precision and exactitude, reproducibility and independence of place and person" and that clinical measurements "staged a central representational technique" of physiological laboratory experiments: "the kymographic method" (ibid: 94).[51]

As a historical event, the introduction of scientific medicine, or *wissenschaftliche Medicin*, into academic and medical discourses changed the general orientation of the discipline of medical science. Contemporaneous physiological and clinical programs were still indebted to a notion of *Bildung*, which meant the cognitive and moral formation of the individual, as it was devised by Romantic reformers at the start of the century. Even the idea of clinical medicine, which had been spreading since the 1820s, stressed the cognitive and moral formation of the practitioner, although here it was exposure to disease in the clinic rather than to life processes in the lab that acted as the key pedagogical element. Only the clinical teacher or laboratory researcher could achieve a true understanding of medicine, which usually also implied a unidirectional relationship between him (all teachers and researchers were male), his knowledge and medical practice.

---

51 The kymograph was a popular physical measuring device invented by the physiologist Carl Ludwig in the 1840s. It measured blood pressure through hydraulic mechanisms and recorded it onto a revolving drum (Bynum 1994: 98f.). Fever measurement imitated this method by recording body temperatures over a period of time onto fever charts (see Hess 1994).

Scientific medicine reconceptualized the relationship between science and medicine in what can be regarded as modern, liberal terms. Its greatest proponent was Rudolf Virchow, the eminent scientist and politician, who popularized the idea in his programmatic writings (Virchow 1847, 1855, 1877). Though Virchow also drew on the idea of exposure to science as a way of instilling the right state of mind into medical professionals, his program deemphasized the Romantic image of the scientist researching in solitude and freedom. He substituted it with an idea of medical science determined by practical procedures and protocols, which were based on the scientific integration of work in the lab and the clinic. He thus removed the elitist idea of science as centered on personal qualities, as with the Romantics. Instead, Virchow reoriented the focus to be more on the methodological and intellectual procedures that enabled arriving at scientific insights for clinical medicine.

Virchow held liberal views and fought on the barricades in the Revolution of 1848/49 (Otis 2007: 148f.). His general concern was with the working-class people of Prussia. He saw "that medicine should be used to reform society, and that it had been created – and should be run – by the practical, hardworking middle class" (ibid: 156). His conception of medical science reflected this attitude. Science was supposed to be employed for finding ways to heal, rather than for only finding natural laws. Additionally, Virchow's program made explicit use of the hospital "working class", i.e., the medical staff. While his contemporaries held on to the Romantic and elitist ideals of the academic professional, for him, just about anybody who knew how research worked could contribute to generating knowledge about disease, without having to be a genuine researcher themselves. Virchow significantly reinvented pathology through his cellular theory and pioneered the field successfully as a modern science. In contrast to his contemporaries, who saw no real use for microscopy in medical science, he emphasized the centrality of a microscopical research culture to study *abnormal* conditions of organic nature. In 1856, the University of Berlin created the first pathological institute in Germany as an epitome to his successful institution-building. He was an astute pathological researcher, studying and naming many important diseases (particularly of the blood), like leukemia and thrombosis (Bynum 1994: 123–127).

Most importantly, however, as a basic concept, scientific medicine was able to maneuver the complicated intellectual and institutional landscape at mid-century between laboratory science and clinical medicine as well as between ideologies of pure and applied science. As Désirée Schauz observes, the fundamental distinction "pure/applied", which organized the scientific system in the nineteenth century, was not set in stone. Although it provided a classification for sorting the hierarchies between and inside scientific disciplines, the labels were "relative" and depended on the respective disciplinary standpoints (Schauz 2020: 197). "The boundary drawing and claims to taking a superior position in the hierarchy of disciplines and for providing the foundation for the subordinate disciplines was quite contested" (ibid: 198). Medicine was commonly construed as an applied science because it increasingly depended on the insights from existing basic science disciplines like biology and chemistry; because it had the express aim of contributing to the practice of healing; and because it had supposedly no body of knowledge of its own. But others defended it as a pure science on the ground of having "the specific nature of disease" as its own unique object of interest (ibid: 197f.). Virchow regarded medical practice as *applied* scientific medicine, which had to study disease close to where it happened, so to speak, rather than arriving at clinical insights from abstract deliberations generated from instrument measurements. At the same time, he was a strong proponent of academic freedom and of the independence of research from any immediate practical ends – a position that was especially evident in his arguments for pathology as an independent science.[52] This combination was something that distinguished Virchow chiefly from his colleagues, both as a clinician and a laboratory scientist.

I. Medicine as an Exact Science – The Physiological Program

When looking back on the publishing history of his journal *Archiv für pathologische Anatomie und Physiologie und klinische Medicin* (which he had been editing since 1847) form his prestigious position as institute head and physician to the German crown in 1877, Virchow recollected that what his generation had above all realized in the past thirty years was that not only physiology but pathology, too, had to be an independent science if medicine was to be genuinely scientific. It did "not suffice to conceive of pathology as applied physiology", he claimed. Instead, it required a "pathological physiology with its proper field of work and independent activity" (Virchow 1958: 149 [1877: 8f.], see also 1849: 18, 1855: 4). As someone who chose his words carefully (Otis 2007: 154), he employed the term "pathological physiology" to at the same time signal his allegiance to the

---

52 This does not mean, however, that he was not able to frame science in the emerging material interests of state and society (Schauz 2020: 216ff.).

physiological tradition of medical science – after all, he had been reared in the lab of the famous physiologist and anatomist Johannes Müller (who was a direct descendent of Romantic medicine) – and to distinguish his approach from that of his contemporaries, who practiced a physicalist approach to physiological questions.

The ill-defined discipline of physiology, which I discussed in the previous chapter, was taking on more defined form around 1850, differentiating into the physicalist approach, scientific anatomy and the biological science of zoology, amongst others (Nyhart 1995). Physicalists aimed at reducing the study of physiological function to the paradigms of physics and chemistry, i.e., to a common set of experimental methods and mathematical techniques.[53] Virchow foregrounded microscopy, which was employed in anatomy, as the central research culture to study the cellular manifestation of disease. Accordingly, acquiring a *habitus* forged through the science of microscopy was a vital element to cultivate the territory of medical science. In giving his retrospect, Virchow also revealed the double conceptual strategy, which he had pursued in the three previous decades: to establish medicine as an *applied science* it required for pathology to be constituted as a *pure science*, which, in turn, would renew and maintain the disciplinary identity of medicine. What were the reasons for him to venture on this path in the 1840s and 1850s?

What the younger Virchow found in the mid-nineteenth century were contrasting efforts to establish medicine according to the sciences of the day, which were, however, threatening to fragment its disciplinary identity. For Virchow it was unquestionable that physiology laid the groundwork for modern-day medicine. But he also saw how science and medical practice were moving in different directions. I will discuss the physiological program and the ideological role of the scientific method further down. It will then become apparent that, though actors accounted for the scientific constitution of the physician on the one side and for a physiological current that operated independently from medicine on the other, it no longer embraced the idea of medical science as a unified and independent discipline. In the earlier days, Virchow claimed, physiology and medicine

---

53 Timothy Lenoir (1997) portrays the group of "organic physics". These were physiological physicists, which formed around Emil du Bois-Reymond, Hermann von Helmholtz, Carl Ludwig and other scientists in the early 1840s. They became known for their bold (yet failed) attempts to remove physiology from the medical faculty and place it in an institutional setting among the theoretical sciences, next to other disciplines such as chemistry and physics to make the field "the natural representative of the progressive movement in science" (ibid: 79).

were interrelated, mutually contributing to each other. Now, the idea of *Wissenschaft* had come to dominate for half a decade: "a concept which is nowhere more developed than in Germany and which has nowhere produced more harm than in medicine" (1958: 29 [Virchow 1847: 7], translation modified). The idea of a pure science of physiology had made the field alien to medicine, so "that medical conceptions [*Anschauungen*] have performed without a physiological basis just as physiology has deprived itself of any medical experience" (ibid: 30 [Virchow 1847: 8], translation modified). He accordingly saw the need to renew the relation between science and medicine, which in his case meant making pathology as a pure science the actual basis for clinical practice, while physiology moved to the background as only the general frame in which medical science happened.

Virchow's conceptual innovations were directed at two fronts: on the one side, he was critiquing a medicine based purely on the institution of the clinic, as it had been developing since the early nineteenth century. On the other, he was also opposing the pretensions of the physiological protagonists, who apparently thought they could solve the riddles of the clinic solely from the induction of biological theories through measurement of organic processes. Physiology was now becoming a hugely popular natural science that acted as a conceptual framework for other sciences with its emerging specialties in medicine and in biology (Hagner 2003, Nyhart 1995). For Virchow, physiology in its current state was an impotent medical science, which, by trying to force its paradigm onto practical medicine, as in the category of physiological medicine, did not succeed in "getting to the point of healing" (ibid.). In his 1877 retrospective, he therefore recalled that the elaborations in the early issues of his *Archiv* "were for the most part directed against the so-called 'rational' movement in medicine and the self-designated 'physiological' school, which had been in full bloom at the time." Although he thought it was an unrewarding task "to push back these currents pursued by keen and industrious men" (1877: 9f.).

What did it mean for Virchow that physiology was an impotent medical science? What characterized the competing programs regarding the relationship between science and medicine? A main feature of the new programs was the introduction of the idea that the causes of disease were governed by natural laws. In this, protagonists followed the physicalist paradigm of physiology that was beginning to develop as an independent science. They wanted to create an approach in which the natural sciences provide the overarching theory for the empirical observations of the clinic. In short, these actors took their model from the *natural* sciences like physics or chemistry, instead of from *medical* sciences like pathology. A look at these natural science programs for medicine will help reveal how they contrasted to Virchow's own idea of scientific medicine.

The programs popular at the time, mentioned by Virchow, were that of "rational medicine" by Jacob Henle and Carl von Pfeufer, who both worked and taught at the University of Heidelberg in the mid-nineteenth century. The other was the program of "physiological medicine" by Wunderlich, Roser and Griesinger, who were initially active in Tübingen. Wunderlich would become professor and director of the university hospital in Leipzig in 1850. What united these different programs in their core was the reduction of the genuine medical science of pathology to versions of physiology, which stressed its natural science features. As Henle programmatically announced in the first volume of his new journal *Zeitschrift für rationelle Medicin* in 1844:

> "The central attribute of rational medicine is that it proceeds from individual facts for which it attempts to find an explanation, and in this physiological and pathological facts have equal values. The final goal is, as far as possible, to trace both back to physical and chemical processes, and in this way to bring these facts under common viewpoints with the phenomena of inorganic nature." (Henle 1844: 31, see also Bleker 1981: 123, Tuchman 1993: 80)

For Henle and Pfeufer, pathology and physiology were merely parts of the same science. They proposed explaining the causal relationships between the pathological phenomena by ultimately making them reducible to an understanding of physics and chemistry. But this also meant degrading the status of disease phenomena, the chief object of pathology, in favor of physiological processes. As Tuchman observes, "for a rational medicine to be successful, [Henle] told his readers over and over again, the notion of disease entities had to be replaced by a definition of disease as nothing more than a deviation from normal physiological processes of life brought about by abnormal conditions" (1993: 78, see also Henle 1844: 15f.). The protagonists of rational medicine had demanded that the names given to illnesses serve merely as "Nomina propria", as labels for a "complex of sensory appearances", and not as concepts for a pathophysiological state itself (Henle 1844: 15, see also Tuchman 1993: 78).

The program of "physiological medicine" by Wunderlich, Roser, and Griesinger saw itself in a similar vein. Protagonists understood their program to stand for medicine as an "empirical and inductive science" that could demand for itself "the same methods as for the exact physical sciences" (Roser/Wunderlich 1842: IIf.). But their pursuit was more radical. Pathological descriptions had no other legitimacy than as "practical makeshifts", an unscientific starting point for investigation into the physiological *qua* physical causes of a diseased body (ibid: XI). While for Henle and von Pfeufer pathological phenomena were as such legitimate objects to be studied and explained physiologically, the core of Wunderlich and his school was to reduce pathology entirely to the language of physicalist physiology. Pathology resembled merely "a tool to be employed in tracing the pathways of disturbed organ function" (Lenoir 1997: 106, see also Hess 1993: 258f.). A manifestation of the physicalist paradigm can be grasped from Wunderlich's specialization in the study of fevers, for which he developed an extensive method of thermometry. He produced charts that recorded the progression of fever in a patient over an extended period of days (figure 4.1.). Variations in temperatures over time, he contended, would allow the clinician to identify individual patterns of disease (Bynum 1994: 138, Hess 1994).

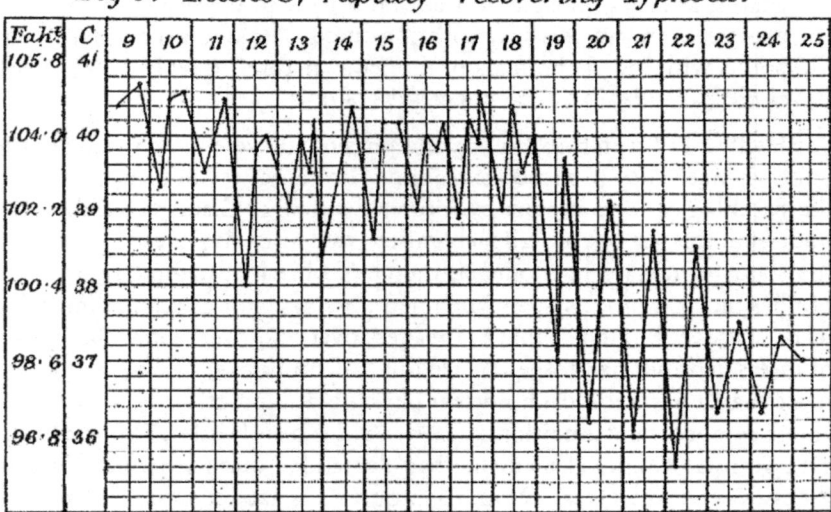

Figure 4.1: *Fever chart (typhoid) from the English edition of Karl August Wunderlich's* On the Temperature in Disease. A Manual of Medical Thermometry. *London 1871. (Source: Wellcome Collection, https://wellcomecollection.org/ works/tk2hrp99, [accessed August 1, 2022]).*

The aim of "physiological medicine" was to oppose the thriving idea of clinical medicine by socializing the medical student in the special physicalist culture of physiology. They wanted to tune his (again, no women in academic medicine at the time) senses to only those phenomena which were measurable with laboratory methods. Roser and Wunderlich had accordingly introduced their new journal, the *Archiv für physiologische Heilkunde*, to readers in 1842 with the assertion that "this one word" – "physiological medicine" – "contains everything that the science [of medicine] possesses, what it demands, and what is essential to it" (1842: I). In the introduction to the second volume in 1843, however, clarifying the assertion made in the prelude, they revealed the radical extent of their program:

> "That physiology control and inform the doctor's entire reasoning, that it purifies his concepts, and forces him, for every pathological fact, to seek the motives for his judgement in the utmost knowledge of the anatomical and functional [=physiological] circumstances of the affected parts – this is the direction in which medicine must strive, and by virtue of which it deserves the name physiological [medicine]." (Roser/Wunderlich 1843: 2)

The proponents of the physiological program wanted to instill a professional *habitus* into the student that comprised schemes of perception, thought and action, which made him see illness inside the patient with the eyes of the "organic physicist", as measurable disturbances of organic function.

Volker Hess has argued that by basing medicine on the model of the natural sciences, and on physicalist physiology in particular, "Wunderlich was fighting for the scientific recognition of the medical clinic" (Hess 1994: 300). Particularly Wunderlich's practice of thermometry was aimed at mimicking the constellation of the experimental natural sciences. Hess shows how the thermometer was framed by Wunderlich to formally embody all criteria, "which at this time could be posed to a measuring experimental setup: it isolated a variable, but measurable physiological function" (Hess 1994: 308). Wunderlich furthermore used the setup to transfer the sort of research questions inherent to physiological experimental methodology to the approach of clinical thermometry, however, replacing scientific values with values for clinical practice (ibid: 309). In other words, rather than consulting an adjacent experimental laboratory, he envisioned the clinic itself to become sort of a lab to study disease in the fashion of the natural sciences (Hess 2010b: 91ff.). This already indicated a move in which the disciplinary identity of medicine would become displaced from the institution of the experimental laboratory. His physicalist approach to measuring fevers already provided the necessary natural science language and an image of objectivity to make the case. As Hess concludes, the rhetoric of objectivity and of methodological autonomy for clinical investigation allowed a broad circle of practicing physicians and readers of the *Archiv für physiologische Heilkunde* "to identify the scientific as well as disciplinary autonomy of the medical clinic with the thermometer and the fever curve" (Hess 1994: 318).

With this framing of clinical medicine as part of the natural sciences, Wunderlich and his allies were opposing a different framing of medicine as scientific, which gained popularity in the 1820s. We do not know very much about the history of university clinics (see Bleker 1995, Hess 2010a,b). But as universities were setting up clinical teaching facilities and receiving access to patients in general hospitals, clinical medicine as a scientific program began to emerge in Germany with the figure of Johann Lucas Schönlein. He was professor of medicine at the University of Würzburg, became director of the medical clinic at the Juliusspital in 1824 and received a chair in Berlin in 1840. Schönlein is founder of what has been called the the Natural Historical School in medicine, which applied classificatory and taxonomical approaches to historical accounts of sickness and the observation of disease in the clinic. He is credited with having systematically integrated the teaching clinic into the concept of academic medicine (Bleker 1981).

In contrast to Wunderlich's natural science approach, Schönlein's idea of clinical medicine was based on an empiricism that combined astute bedside observation with the historical study of disease. Schönlein deemed clinical medicine "scientific" because of its natural-historical methodology. Using a comparative method, doctors' past accounts of sicknesses and symptoms were to be combined with meticulous records of individual patient histories, marking how diseases unfolded temporally and spatially in the individual and in society (Schönlein 1929: 7f., see also Bleker 1981: 71–80, Hess 1993: 238–242). His systematization and classification of disease was furthermore aided by physical and chemical practices. Clinical medicine had been helping itself with the newest scientific and clinical technologies, which complemented the natural historical descriptions with indications of organ damage by adding "a 'physiological' viewpoint" (Hess 1993: 249, see also Hess 1995: 106ff., Bynum 1994: 30–46). Percussion, auscultation, microscopic and chemical analysis had become popular techniques to study disease in the hospital and clinic since the early decades of the century.[54] Clinical teachers like Schönlein therefore maintained small laboratories to run routine diagnostic tests and to perform auxiliary research (Hess 2010b: 97f.). The empirical description of the Natural Historical School resulted in combining symptoms into specific disease patterns, with their disease progression and transformation. Thereby Schönlein's and his school's clinical method gave the rather abstract phenomenon of sickness of former ages a concrete clinical definition in the modern sense.

Schönlein was convinced that previous generations of medical thinkers, especially the Romantics, had distorted the study of disease through their rational speculations. Thereby they created a distinction between theory and practice that harmed the idea of practical medicine. In his inaugural address as professor in Würzburg in 1819, he claimed:

> "All of natural science [*Naturkunde*] was a strong tree when its golden fruit, medicine, appeared. An unfortunate methodology has teared this golden fruit from the living stem in newer times and, through the absolute contrast of theory and practice, twisted nature into un-nature. To compensate for this unnatural [and] mindless opposition [between theory and practice], to show and to prove that theory and practice are one and the same, that they are identical, is the one and only task of the clinic" (Schönlein 1929: 5).

To the speculative and rationalistic approach of the Romantics, Schönlein opposed the clinical method. He was questioning how practical advantages could come from abstract speculations, from philosophical models and representations of biological processes generated away from the actual place where disease happened – in the patient's body. To identify medical theory with practice meant that both had to be founded on the same institution. As Schönlein contended, the clinical method was supposed to account for both the practical and theoretical side of medicine (Bleker 1981: 53). It meant that the treatment of patients and the study of the specific and universal features of disease went hand in hand.

A true experience of disease was therefore only possible in the clinic, which allowed for systematic and controlled observation. Quoting one of Schönlein's students, Hess accordingly remarks that the central idea of the clinical method was that "the clinic 'takes the sickbed as the standpoint from which it scrutinizes all other branches of science for what they can offer it for the ultimate end of healing. All beams of science result in this

---

54 The "breakthrough" event in this respect was the invention of the stethoscope and of the technique of auscultation by Laennec in 1819 (Reiser 1979: 23–44).

center'" (1995: 108f.). Students were accordingly taught to make careful bedside observations of individual patients, to record these observations and use them for making prognosis and therapy. Additionally, however, they were encouraged to use these meticulous reports to ponder on the general causes of specific diseases in humankind, next to the individual causes in a certain patient (Bleker 1981: 55f.).

> "This being next and after each other [*Neben- und Aufeinandersein*] of disease, researching how they have grown apart, affords the physician, who does not locate the highest of his art in the technical and in writing prescriptions, a high, [and] not only scientific interest. Because in this way he finds types of disease [*Krankheitsformen*] in nature next to each other, which are far apart in our textbooks; he sees a common bond between things, which were presented to him as highly heterogeneous and different" (Schönlein 1929: 9).

Schönlein was convinced that "just as in the other teachings of the natural sciences" – with which he meant natural history – also in medicine, "a natural systematization [of disease] is possible" (ibid.).

II. The Ideology of Methodology in Mid-Nineteenth-Century Germany

Schönlein had the same aim as Wunderlich – to argue for the scientific status and disciplinary autonomy of the medical clinic. But both programs did so under vastly different ideologies. These differences were revealed in the role and the status of the natural sciences for medicine, the image of the truly scientific physician and the right methodology to apply to research and teaching. The natural sciences for Schönlein were moulded after the comparative and taxonomic practices of the natural historian, while for Wunderlich the experimental and quantifying approaches of physics acted as a model. For the image of the physician, this resulted in conflicting ideals about the appropriate cognitive and moral qualities. Schönlein's doctors had to be meticulous observers, attentive to the development of disease, its history and the improvement or deterioration of the patient under treatment. Wunderlich's doctors were also meticulous observers, but of the variables and swings in his measuring devices, and of the significance this had for understanding biological processes. The practices and virtues being taught in a clinic-based medical education were those that Hess has aptly described as forming the "clinical doctor", and not so much the natural science-minded physician or the future medical scientist (Hess 1993: 18, 1995: 108, s. also Tuchman 1993: 66).

Historian Johanna Bleker has suggested that the structural differences between Schönlein's clinical and Wunderlich's physiological program was not as great as the polemics they exchanged might imply. In fact, she argues, "the manner in which the physiological current wants to investigate the essence of disease has a remarkable similarity with Schönlein's approach" (1981: 117). We can take this observation as an indication of the playing field on which both schools fought over primacy in academic medicine, namely, that of ideology. More generally, competing ideologies surfaced especially in debates over methodology in the context of education around the mid-nineteenth century. I want to include this to also mean debates over scientific and clinical methods. As Phillips shows, controversies over methods in Germany pertained to questions of professional and anthropological characteristics. "*Methodologie* dealt extensively with personal qualities," she notes, "the concrete competencies and character traits necessary to practice a given science or profession" (Phillips 2012: 238). As she demonstrates, though, rhetoric of the scientific method was foremost used by actors to discursively distinguish the human and the natural sciences. Nevertheless, we can gain some insight for academic medicine more specifically and how the clinical method and the scientific method were opposed here.

Advocates of the scientific method aimed at presenting a refined concept of *Bildung* in the mid-nineteenth century (Phillips 2012: 239ff., Schauz 2020: 224f.). They stressed the epistemological particularity of the natural sciences in contrast to that of the humanities. As we saw earlier, whereas neo-humanists advocated that "the classical curriculum was the best preparation for boys whose lives would be devoted to *Wissenschaft*", the "German *Naturfoscher*" was keen on showing that "the natural sciences had their own distinct epistemological contribution to make" and that they "provided skills different from those that could be gained studying books" (ibid: 230). They used qualities such as a refined sensory perception, critical observation and hands-on experience as markers for a pedagogical ideal that stressed practical-intellectual purposes, but nevertheless understood the natural sciences to constitute a unified body of knowledge (ibid: 245, see also Bonner 1995a: 236ff.). Stated differently, for these actors, the scientific method represented a reformed notion of the moral and intellectual source that would now mold the elite researcher, just as *Bildung* formed its equivalent in previous decades. As Phillips furthermore notes, "the idea that refined sensory perception was the hallmark of the *Naturforscher* (and by extension the medical doctor) was a commonplace in introductory textbooks, both in the natural sciences proper and in medicine" (ibid: 249). Thus, by stressing the superiority of the skills acquired through training in the method, it worked rhetorically to defend the natural sciences curriculum against the humanist curriculum.

In the case of academic medicine, actors also stressed the epistemological particularity of the scientific and clinical method. Reference to either the clinical or the scientific method worked for protagonists to emphasize different cognitive and moral qualities in the academic physician. Moreover, it functioned to map different relationships between the institutions of the clinic and experimental science. Wunderlich wanted students to be trained to see medicine through the eyes of physiology as an exact physical science, while Schönlein's students were to see it through the rich history and system of disease. For Schönlein, the natural sciences employed in the clinical context merely constituted aids, because of their reduced role to diagnostics and analysis. Wunderlich's program was built on the skills and qualities students received in laboratory training, although it depended on other laboratories to provide such training. In the eyes of physiological contemporaries, therefore, clinical medicine deprived the medical discipline of its exact science identity, by delegating the laboratory to the status of a handmaiden. In reaction, Wunderlich and his allies tried to very publicly make a central place for physiology and the method of the natural sciences (see figure 4.2). For this purpose, they debased the epistemological peculiarities of clinical medicine and its method. The dirty manner of the debates again suggests that the playing field was that of ideology and not of scientific facts or proofs.

The central critique levelled against Schönlein's Natural Historical School was the supposed reliance on an ontological understanding of disease. Wunderlich and his conspirators very publicly accused Schönlein and his followers of an irresponsible adherence to the outdated idea of disease entities (Bleker 1981: 114–126). In effect, this was meant to suggest that Schönlein and his allies were still adhering to premodern and antiquated medical philosophies. The *Archiv für physiologische Heilkunde* turned into a collection of polemics against the Natural Historical School in the half decade after its inauguration. Protagonists wondered "how one could tolerate the fact that its inventor [Schönlein] claims [to have a] monopoly on an exclusive-natural scientific medicine" (Roser/Wunderlich 1841: X, see also Bleker 1981: 116). As Bleker argues, though, Wunderlich and his followers only feinted the radical opposition between their own and Schönlein's program. Schönlein had made it unmistakable that the idea of disease entities acted merely as a methodological device for the empirical study of sickness (Schönlein 1929: 7). He simply demanded of his students that every disease ought to be treated as *if it were* a concrete object. "Thereby it becomes very clear that he is not at all asserting that disease are concrete objects, but only that one needs to study them as if they were entities sui generis. This demand has nothing to do with his general definition of illness [sic]" (Bleker 1981: 55, see also Hess 1993: 250).

But instead of philosophical, actors rather had institutional axes to grind. By implying that Schönlein's clinical method conveyed thinking in an antiquated fashion, proponents were emphasizing the role of training in the experimental laboratory sciences. Their main worry was to legitimize a natural sciences-based education, so that future doctors approach problems in the clinic with the appropriate mindset and skills (Bleker 1981: 124f.). At the University of Heidelberg, the proponents of "rational medicine", Henle and von Pfeufer, introduced extensive practical training in various scientific methods into the curriculum in the 1840s that would expose medical students to a natural sciences environment (Tuchman 1993: 72–77). And Wunderlich, too, made practical clinical training in Leipzig mandatory that required physiological reasoning and scientific methodology (Lenoir 1997: 123–127). Rhetorical emphasis on scientific methodology was a way to articulate the essential features that training in the scientific laboratory provided to the medical student over their training in the clinic.

The effects of degrading clinical medicine in favor of the physiological approach, however, had far-reaching structural implications for medical science as a discipline. Wunderlich's program split the originally unitary idea of a discipline as composed of research and teaching into two, where the teaching remained in the institution of the laboratory, since it required the skills of experimental sciences, while the research part was moved to the clinic. This separation plaid more into the hands of those medical scientists who were beginning to remove themselves from medical practice, like the "organic physicists", rather than for those seeking to make the clinic a sort of a natural sciences laboratory. Historian Timothy Lenoir argues that the famous physiologist Carl Ludwig capitalized on the ideological understanding of the scientific method. The establishment of Ludwig's institute at the University of Leipzig in 1869 (the first of the major physiological institutes to be founded in Germany in the late-nineteenth century), according to Lenoir, needs to be seen as the result of his strategic bargaining for material gain for his enterprise. Employing the rhetoric of the scientific method, Ludwig rendered the science of physiology "serviceable to the practical needs of clinical medicine", to secure funding for his cause of strengthening the discipline of physiology. "This did not imply giving up the disinterested pursuit of knowledge. Rather, it meant coordinating scientific research with the material interests of the state" (Lenoir 1997: 129, see also Kremer 2009: 355f.). We can now better understand what this entailed – namely, framing the pure science laboratory as a training ground for clinicians.

Lenoir also shows how Wunderlich structurally prepared the advent of Ludwig and his research institute: "A more harmonious fit than that between Ludwig's perspective on physiology and Wunderlich's program for physiological medicine", he argues, "could scarcely be imagined" (ibid: 127). Ludwig pursued a physiological research program that had little to do with clinical practice (ibid: 107ff.). Training in the scientific method, however, which he provided in his laboratory, was for students that went on to become practicing physicians. In sociological terms, he was rearing a tribe for settlement on a foreign territory, namely, the clinic. They were not being prepared for medical research (ibid: 115). In a way, Ludwig and Wunderlich thus represented two separated disciplinary programs in which one depended unilaterally on the other. However, judging from the degree of institutionalization that followed, we need to consider that Ludwig's scientific program superseded that of Wunderlich.

III. Rudolf Virchow's Program of Scientific Medicine

Virchow emphasized medicine as an *applied science* in part to distinguish his idea from the likes of Wunderlich (and Ludwig), who were more interested in the methods of physiology as a pure science. For him, the fact that medicine had to be an applied science did not reduce its status among the other sciences, though. On a general level, the designation placed his concept of scientific medicine in the realm of pursuits dedicated to the common good, just as technology was beginning to be framed as the result of a knowledge transfer from science, which led to general improvements (Schauz/Lax 2018: 67). Furthermore, in medical discourses concretely, the label worked to elevate his concept of pathology as a full-blown academic science within the context of the medical discipline. If medical practice was applied scientific medicine, then pathology laid the theoretical foundations for this purpose and therefore constituted the chief science of scientific medicine and the medical discipline (Benaroyo 1998).

Virchow argued that this constellation would restore the central objective of medical science, which was to be able to heal sick patients. "Virchow wanted a renewal of medicine from the inside out – from the morgue and the microscope to the wards – and he focused on clinical practice. To him, the bottom line of any epistemological strategy was its value to the suffering patient" (Otis 2007: 146). His contemporaries seemed to have exchanged this objective for purely scientific pursuits (through the Romantic influence). Whether it was investigating life processes in the physiological laboratory or studying disease in the clinic using physical measuring techniques – in both cases protagonists seemed to follow the primacy of scientific research rather than that of healing patients. But there is need for qualification.

Virchow was just as much a proponent of scientific freedom and research autonomy as his contemporaries in physiology were. As already mentioned, he was a liberal and concerned with Prussia's working-class. But it needs to be recognized how this fact reflected in his ideas about medical science specifically. Although Virchow held simultaneous appointments in the University of Berlin and the Charité hospital throughout his career, he had little interest in medical practice beyond the routine inspections he was obliged to. As Cay-Rüdiger Prüll notes, in fact, Virchow "was not very successful in therapy"; and when making his ward rounds, he examined patients like a clinician should, but appeared to be more interested in the manifestations of disease that would only become visible during autopsy (2000: 97f.). This attitude was not unusual. Hermann von Helmholtz became professor of physiology at the University of Heidelberg in 1858. As Tuchman notes, he showed scant interest in practical medicine. In the decades following his appointment, he "remained aloof from routine drill conducted in his laboratory. [...] Helmholtz distanced himself even further from his 'medical' duties by requiring his assistant to teach his courses in microscopical anatomy, justifying this by his lack of histological knowledge and his tendency to get headaches" (Tuchman 1993: 161). What distinguished Virchow's program from that of his contemporaries, however, was not the general orientation towards medicine, but only the research orientation of medical science. Wunderlich and the physicalists (like Ludwig and Helmholtz later in the century) were seeking to understand the natural laws of biological processes. Virchow, in contrast, was aiming to arrive at scientific principles for clinical practice by directly studying disease according to the paradigm of the natural sciences (I will explain this shortly).

Clearly, Virchow saw some confusion over what a science-based medicine meant to his contemporaries. There was obviously no "core agreement" on the idea of scientific medicine among him and his rivals, as historians of German medicine tend to believe. Virchow introduced readers to his new *Archiv* in 1847 with an important plea to end the confusion: "When speaking of scientific medicine, at the present time," he claimed, "it is highly necessary to come to agreement concerning the meaning of the words" (1958: 26 [Virchow 1847: 3]). He programmatically differentiated between "practical medicine" and "scientific medicine" in the text to signal that his program meant more than the relationship between physiology and clinical practice:

> "Ever since we recognized that diseases are neither self-subsistent, circumscribed, autonomous organisms, nor entities which have forced their way into the body, nor parasites rooted on it, but that they represent only the course of physiological phenomena under altered conditions – ever since this time the goal of therapy has to be the maintenance or the reestablishment of normal physiological conditions.
> The actual accomplishment or, put more precisely, the striving for an actual accomplishment, of this aim comprises the task of practical medicine.
> Scientific medicine, for its part, has as its object the investigation of those altered conditions which characterize the diseased body or various ailing organs, the identification of abnormalities in the phenomena of life as they occur under specifically altered conditions, and finally, the discovery of means for abolishing these abnormal conditions" (ibid: 26f. [1847: 3f.]).

While practical medicine was thus defined as restoring or maintaining the normal life functions in the patient, the actual province of scientific medicine was pathology and therapy, and not physiology. The point of scientific medicine is the acquisition of knowledge about altered life conditions, and of the means to neutralize these conditions. Of course, maintaining the normal state necessarily also presupposed a knowledge of normal functions. Virchow was implying those keen and industrious men, who tried appropriating pathology with the concepts of physicalist physiology. Committed principally to the pure science ideal, however, "the most recent developments in medicine" made it "appear as if this had hardly anything to do" at all with the matter of healing (ibid.). He programmatically proclaimed that the sciences of pathology and therapy could only be constructed from inside of the institution of practical medicine, "and we dispute the right of any discipline not itself rooted in the observation of diseased life to share in the interpretation of its phenomena" (ibid: 31f. [Virchow 1847: 10], translation modified). The possibility to observe disease, as he saw it, rested equally within the pathological laboratory, where diseased bodies were dissected, and the clinic, where sick patients were treated. As will become clear in the following, in a crucial sense, his program offered a sort of middle ground between the competing factions of clinical and physiological medicine: by integrating the institutions of the laboratory and the clinic equally, instead of only relating them hierarchically. "Poised between the university and hospital, between *Wissenschaft* and the clinical bustle of the Berlin Charité, Virchow through his [pathological] institute stood ready to investigate the productions of each in the terms of the other" (Maulitz 1978: 170).

a. The Science of Pathology

One central part of Virchow's strategy was to renew the scientific basis of medicine. As I showed above, he regarded physiology as no longer appropriate for the task of founding medical practice. It was not enough to instruct doctors as physiologists and send them out into the clinic in the hopes that they, upon contact with the sick patient, would deduce the right methods of action from the laws of organic nature they had observed in the lab and/or the clinic. For this reason, he claimed that pathology was a pure and full-blown science laying the foundations for any knowledge of practical medicine to be constructed. In his 1877 retrospective, he proclaimed:

> "Now that the work is done, we need to remain aware [of the fact] that the emancipation of pathology, the ennoblement of pathology to the rank of a natural science, requires that pathologists keep their independence, that they do not allow any external science [*fremde Wissenschaft*] to introduce their hypotheses readily into pathology; and that they do not let the latter be forced back into the position of merely an applied science" (Virchow 1877: 9).

The founding of scientific medicine on the science of pathology was not simply intended to displace physiology; the intention was rather to mend the purported impotency of the discipline, which physiology had caused in relation to medical matters. Virchow recalled Bacon's famous dictum "*scientia est potentia*" in his programmatic introduction to the *Archiv* in 1847. He honored his physiological contemporaries for their advancement of scientific knowledge, but in a scathing critique that was unmistakably directed at Wunderlich and the other physicalist physiologists, he claimed that "this is no real knowledge, which is not also able [to perform] what it knows; and what sort of precarious ability it is, not knowing what it does!" (Virchow 1847: 5).

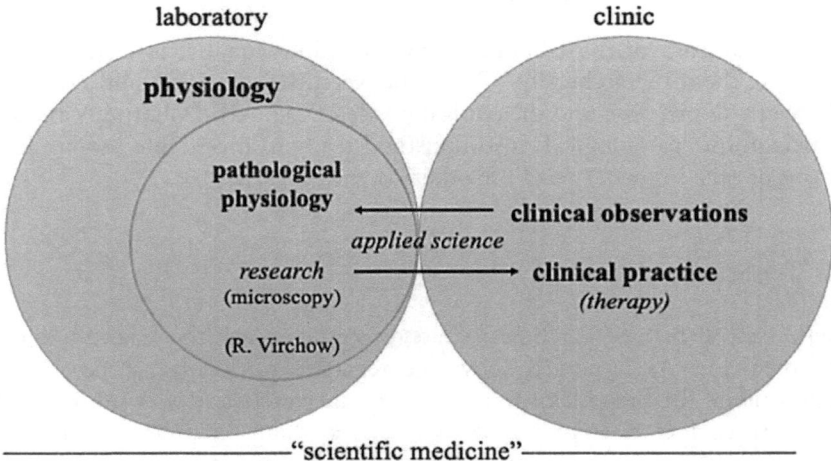

Figure 4.2:   Schema of the structural relationship between laboratory and clinic as well as research and clinical practice in Virchow's idea of "scientific medicine" (my depiction).

As Virchow reflected in 1877, his efforts in the past thirty years had been "to introduce a scientific language into medicine" that would prevent newly found insights from becoming tarnished "by sudden ideas, by improper generalizations, [or] by the tendency to figuratively translate concepts" (1877: 4). In other words, medical scientists and practitioners had to desist speaking in the language of abstract laws and physiological theories and start employing a language with which to comprehend the concrete phenomena clinicians encountered in their everyday routine. "Pathology, which had once consisted of speculations about humors and solids in general, and then moved to the organs and tissues, seemed now to come to a final basis on the ultimate cellular components of organic structure" (Benaroyo 1998: 115). As part of the natural sciences, it would introduce a common conceptual ground for medical research and practice into the medical discipline that would allow the orientation of both upon each other, instead of the one-way direction from physiology to practical medicine engrained in the competing programs. It therefore entailed setting up a cultural foundation that would speak equally to the pathologist as a researcher and the clinician as a practitioner. Initially, Virchow named it "pathological physiology" in 1847, but later in the 1850s refined it famously to constitute his "cellular pathology" (Virchow 1855). A central feature of pathological physiology was therefore to know what practical medicine was void of and what had to be investigated in order to improve its scientific foundation: "Pathological physiology receives its questions in part from pathological anatomy, and from practical medicine; it generates answers in part from observation at the sickbed, and therefore is part of the clinic, and in part from animal experiment" (Virchow 1958: 37 [1847: 16f.], translation modified). Medical knowledge, in other words, relied on the combination of close clinical observation, animal experiment and systematic autopsy aided by histology and chemical analysis (Prüll 2000: 91, Otis 2007: 146).

I will illustrate the functioning of the conceptual space using the example of Virchow's cellular pathology. The development and institutional consequences of Virchow's pathological theory are well known (e.g., Maulitz 1978, Schmiedebach 1992). My purpose here is only to provide a general outline regarding the production of a scientific culture for the shared orientation of scientific and medical action. First, I need to clarify some names, though. From current standpoints, Virchow's cellular pathology would be considered as pathological anatomy and histology (see figure 4.3), that is, a subfield of anatomy, although when Virchow published his famous piece on the theory as an editorial in his *Archiv* in 1855, he saw it as a first culmination in his intention of "founding a *pathological physiology*" and not anatomy (Virchow 1855: 6). However, the combined approaches of anatomy and physiology were only starting to become institutionally separated in the 1850s (Nyhart 1995: 84ff.). Thus, Virchow's ideas drew on the shared anatomical-physiological tradition that emerged at the start of the century, and became exemplified in Johannes Müller, though his emphasis on anatomical methods was clearly intended to separate his approach from that of physicalist physiology. However, his employment of the term physiology made it clear that he still saw himself indebted to the scientific tradition of physiology, which emerged with Reil and matured with Müller and his pupils. His article on cellular pathology was followed by a book in 1858, with the same name: *Cellular Pathology*, comprising lectures he held at his pathological institute in Berlin.

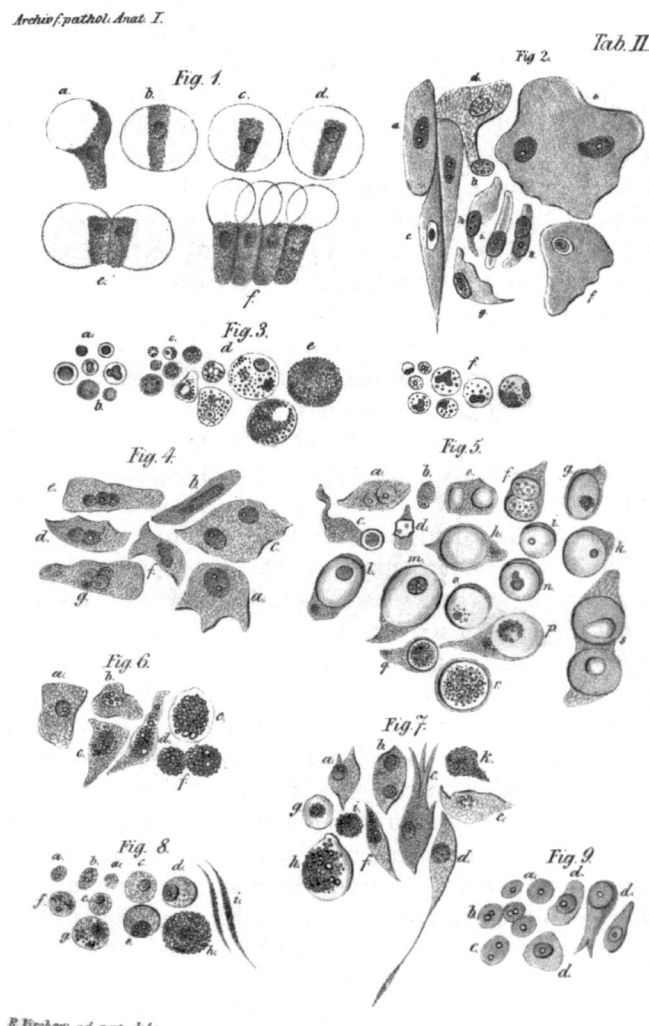

Figure 4.3: *Different cancerous cells illustrated by Virchow from microscopic investigations and printed in the first issue of his Archiv. (Source: Rudolf Virchow. 1847. Zur Entwicklungsgeschichte des Krebs nebst Bemerkungen über Fettbildung im thierischen Körper und pathologische Resorption.* Archiv für pathologische Anatomie und Physiologie und für klinische Medizin *1(1), p. 206 https://commons.wikimedia.org/wiki/File:Virchow-cell.jpg [accessed August 1, 2022]).*

Second, the development of the achromatic compound microscope in the 1830s allowed investigators for the first time to observe living tissue at high resolutions over comparatively long periods without straining their eyes. As a result, Müller's student Theodor Schwann revealed that animal organisms are composed of cells or of structures produced by cells, after Matthias Schleiden had previously proven the case for plants (Harris 1999: 94–105). Virchow applied a modified version of this theory to pathology, which stated that all tissue – diseased and normal – originate within the cell from physical and chemical mechanisms (Virchow 1855: 15).[55] Virchow constructed his idea of pathology on a "conception of the human body as an organized cell state, a social system of continuous development, in which each microscopic cellular unit performed its parts" (Benaroyo 1998: 115). Accordingly, the theory holds that every illness can be traced back to disturbances of living cells, causing large parts of the "cell state" to deteriorate, and it required that "the physiology of pathological developments be pursued hand in hand with the history of normal developments" (Virchow 1855: 14). In short, Virchow's theory replaced the idea of organic lesions as the cause for functional impairments with that of disturbed cell growth, that is, as anatomical aberrations causing organic functions to fail.

The advantage of this concept over those of his medical competition was that it allowed to center scientific medicine on the science of microscopy, which could – literally – provide a common focal point tangible for both science and medicine, compared to the rather abstract biological processes only inferred to from work with physiological measuring devices. "Disease processes," according to Virchow, "were to be studied by medical microscopists with pathological training" (Maulitz 1978: 169). Thus, for him, the microscope constituted an agent of true reform in medicine in an age when anatomy was only starting to become part of the natural sciences in its own right (Virchow 1855: 8, see also Nyhart 1995: 80–90). While the instrument was increasingly being used as a diagnostic aid, only few had actually learned to *think* microscopically in medicine, Virchow asserted; and he demanded that not the use of the instrument as a practical tool, but the epistemic virtues of the science become the foundation for pathology and therapy, that is, "scientific medicine" (ibid: 7, 38).[56] As the pathologist

---

55 The famous dictum connected with Virchow's theory is the "*Omnis cellula e cellula*" (1855: 23). Historian Henry Harris provides a portray of Virchow's controversial role in the formation and spread of cell theory (1999: 132–137).

56 Henle had both used the instrument for scientific study while working with Müller in Berlin, and later in Heidelberg taught the technique to his medical

would thus become accustomed to "the finer construction of the body by his own perception [*Anschauung*]", and subsequently interpret experiences "in accordance with this conception [*Anschauung*]", it would ultimately enable the practitioner to "thinking microscopically" (ibid: 100 [1855: 38f.], translation modified). Bynum aptly notes that instead of recording the progression of symptoms or measuring biological processes, "microscopy encouraged doctors to think about the dynamics of disease, about the genesis of lesions rather than their gross, end-stage structures" (1994: 123).

To illustrate, Virchow drew an analogy between the role of the microscope for biology – and by extension pathology – and the meaning of the telescope in astronomy (ibid: 16f.). Naturally, it was indispensable that an astronomer knew how to handle a telescope, Virchow argued. But his objects of interest – the sun, moon, stars, the milky way and nebulas – are also visible with the unaided eye. However, compared to the simple observer, the astronomer has a different perception of these objects. Even without the direct aid of his instrument, he resolves the same moon, stars and nebulas visible in the night sky into a large number of telescopic images every time he *thinks* astronomically. Equally, under the microscope, "everything that lives is dissolved into tiny elements, not all too small that their presence cannot be recognized with the naked eye, to be sure, but possessing a structure so fine that a clear understanding of it is completely impossible without a microscopic conception [*Anschauung*]" (Virchow 1958: 82 [1855: 17], trans. mod.). In short, the pathologist – and by extension the clinician – needs to acquire a professional *habitus* premised on the science of microscopy.

Virchow wanted to give science and medicine an idea of disease as an empirical and tangible object. The different visual representations of the same disease in the pathological laboratory and in the clinic allowed his concepts to transgress disciplinary and institutional boundaries. Thrombosis and cancerous tissues now occupied a shared space, rather than being sicknesses, which derived from abstract physiological deliberations; they functioned as what in STS discourse has become known as "boundary objects" (Star/Griesmer 1989). This point is important, since in the debates around biomedicine, the aligning of the cultures of science and medicine is regarded as a unique feature of medicine in the post-war era. Keating and Cambrosio (2003), for instance, have influentially called biomedicine

---

students (Nyhart 1995: 84, Tuchman 1993: 57f., 76f.). But his approach was nonetheless physicalist, that is, not requiring students to 'think' microscopically, but rather in physical laws.

a "hybrid practice" of biology and medicine. Informed by "new entities and events", which have emerged with post-war molecular biology, biomedicine allows to coordinate knowledge and action of normal biology and pathology, without reducing the one to the other (Keating/Cambrosio 2004: 368, s. also 2003: 76). However, the objects identified by Virchow's pathologists were already simultaneously plastic enough to orient actions individually, both in medical science and practice, but also stable enough to suggest a common identity across the boundary of both institutions. As a result, pathological physiology presented the discipline of medicine as better oriented towards practical medicine and thereby justified its medical identity.

b. A Science of Therapy

As I illustrated above, the programs of Virchow's contemporaries still adhered to the Romantic image of the scientist as someone who is part of an elite and labors in solitude. Accordingly, their concern was with instilling the right cognitive and moral constitution in the student, which, by extension, would also qualify him as a physician (there were generally no woman doctors until the end of the nineteenth century). The protagonists of physiological medicine thought it sufficient, to infer the instructions for clinical actions from the natural laws governing organic life. In their ideological understanding of the scientific method, they believed clinical problems could be solved by sending practitioners into the clinic, who were scientifically educated, but ultimately had no way to assess the theories for their actions other than the crude means of trial and error.

Wunderlich published an article in 1845 titled "The relation of pathological medicine to medical practice" (*Das Verhältniss der physiologischen Medicin zur ärztlichen Praxis*), which made clear how his program still depended on the traditional image of the physician. It shows how he had no formalized concept for therapy other than the quasi-religious beliefs in the capabilities of a doctor and his natural sciences *Bildung*. After lengthy expositions about the different traditions and methods for diagnosis and medical theory-building, chemical analysis and physical examination, Wunderlich draws a preliminary conclusion: "Only after a thorough examination [*Erforschung*] of the objective facts [*Thatbestand*] has occurred, can we speak of considering the individual case theoretically, combining the elements found through analysis into a whole of inner relationships and connecting it to the causes" (Wunderlich 1845: 11). Immediately after, he makes the strange remark that in many cases "this happens by itself". What does he mean? The answer follows in a climatic praise of the physiological physician, which could not have been phrased more emphatically by a true Romantic: "Only the physiological physician knows his task, only the physiological physician, endowed with the necessary knowledge and skills, is able to meet it: only he can know what his patient lacks, only he can judge a clinical case [*Krankheitsfall*], only he will be able to prescribe a rational therapy plan [*vernunftgemäß Heilplan*]" (ibid: 11f.).

Clearly, for Wunderlich everything in academic medicine centered on the scientific doctor and his enlightened spirit. From a scientific standpoint, however, this approach left therapy far behind. True, Virchow was similarly stressing personal and professional qualities with his insistence on the research culture of microscopy and cellular pathology. Later in his career, he would more emphatically emphasize the role of the natural sciences for moral education to counter the overwhelmingly material connotations associated with scientific progress (Schauz 2020: 223). But unlike his contemporaries, Virchow saw the scientific method not primarily as ideological. For him it meant more than sending people with the right cognitive and moral qualities to practice medicine. The method rather provided a practical rigor that could be extended beyond the laboratory to integrate it with the clinic (Benaroyo 1998). In this sense, it enabled a conceptualization of medical practice that was uniquely modern and adapted to the young aspiring industrial state (compared to Wunderlich's Romantic connotations) because it centered the idea of science on actual research practices.

After mid-century, reforms of higher education made science available to a broad spectrum of students and the general orientation of scientific training had shifted. While science was still an elitist pursuit during the Romantic Era, students in the second half of the nineteenth century underwent scientific training to acquire a mindset and skills that would enable them to actively partake in the industrial and economic growth of society. In the early century, only students who seemed promising for pursuing a career in the natural sciences received thorough laboratory training; now scientific methodology was presented as essential equipment for all professionals pursuing careers in the vastly expanding industrial society. As a result, an education in laboratory techniques became to be available equally to all the students enrolled into the course of medicine (Lenoir 1997: 98–104, see also Coleman 1988: 39f.). "Like computers today," Arleen Tuchman argues, "the scientific method in the nineteenth century provided an instrument for teaching school children and college students not only specific skills but also a particular way of approaching, defining, tackling, and solving problems" (1993: 7). She, like others, considers the emergence of training in the methodology of the natural sciences on a broad scale around 1850 as "a tool for the democratization of medicine", since it allowed to replace "talent and intuition" with "routine methods" (ibid: 83, see also Hess 1993: 264).

Virchow adhered to this liberal idea of the scientific method as characterized by routine and instrumental aspects. In his essay on cellular pathology, he accordingly argued for a pragmatic understanding of science in medicine:

"It does not matter at all whether someone is a professor of clinical medicine or of theoretical pathology, whether he is a practitioner or a hospital physician, if only he possesses material for observation. In addition, it is not of decisive significance whether he confronts an overwhelming or a modest amount of material, if only he understands how to exploit it" (Virchow 1958: 77 [1855: 11]).

This meant that the practitioner "must be in a position to put the right questions and to find the right methods for answering them", making practical use of scientific methodology wherever the questions demanded it (ibid.). This was already a clear rejection of the elitist Romantic ideal of the solitary and free scientist. The actions of practical medicine had to be assessed scientifically in the institution of the clinic and by whomever was practically capable to perform such a task.

Virchow's pragmatic understanding of the scientific method was connected to his liberal political views and it reflected in how he conceptualized the institution of the clinic. A more pragmatic understanding of scientific methodology will also come to play a significant part in early-twentieth-century discourses of scientific medicine in the United States, as I discuss in the next chapter. There, however, it was framed within a general ideology of social progress. The clear aim of Virchow's concept of scientific medicine, in contrast, was to heal patients, who in a large part derived from the working middle class. But again, there is need for qualification: the chief way Virchow saw that he could help patients was through *science*. To come to scientific pronouncements on therapy, it required to study disease in patients. Therefore, similar to Wunderlich, patients constituted a crucial research object. "Virchow's writing demonstrates why, for him, clinical findings and theories of disease were inseparable. In his view, patients were the source of knowledge just as they were the reason for its creation" (Otis 2007: 155).

The liberal political understanding extended also to the realm of academic professions and to the divisions of scientific work as such, which separates Virchow's pragmatism from his contemporaries' Romanticism-infused values. The scientific method was not confined to the natural sciences laboratory, nor was it the sole province of the natural scientist. Instead, it could be encountered just about everywhere where scientific issues were being pursued. For Virchow it was evident that "the practicing physician and the clinician", who in a sense constituted the hospital "working class", had unique access to the experience of diseases and their treatment. This fact had to be acknowledged by integrating these roles into the process of scientific study. As the clinical tradition of Schönlein had shown: "all the others, who do not stand by the sickbed, can at best annunciate points of view, perhaps direct the investigation, and keep a critical eye on the principles of therapy [...]" (ibid: 56 [Virchow 1849: 22]). The institution of the clinic was crucial, in other words, because it allowed to scientifically observe the practice of medicine in action; how specific therapies worked in the case of certain pathological conditions, how the state of patients improved or worsened. "Only from this time on will therapy begin to develop like a natural science," Virchow claimed, "for all of the natural sciences begin with empirical observation" (ibid: 57 [Virchow 1849: 23]). In correspondence, the role of the clinician was stressed as that of a practitioner and researcher. Stated differently, the task of the clinician was to gather therapeutic data and evidence of medical treatments. This could be achieved by employing scientific methodology, using it, just as in the laboratory, to control the observations made in the clinic. Hence, Virchow saw that "appointment to a clinic is in our time such an immensely important task because the clinician of our days has to be not only a scientific practitioner," as the physiological proponents asserted, "but also a researcher, an observer" of clinical phenomena (Virchow 1847: 5).

What exactly did Virchow's pragmatic understanding of the scientific method entail? And how was it different from the ideological usage? Virchow chose his words carefully to avoid being grouped too closely with his main physiological opponents. He titled the programmatic essays that appeared thirty years apart, assessing the state of affairs in academic medicine from his respective viewpoints, "Standpoints in Scientific Medicine" (*Ueber die Standpunkte in der wissenschaftlichen Medicin*) (1847, 1877, see also Virchow 1958: 26–39, 142–150). But he also used the unabbreviated adjective *naturwissenschaftlich*, which signifies the modern English "scientific", throughout the running text of his essays (Virchow 1847: 6, 9, 15, 1849: 5,

7, 9, 23, 1855: 3, 11, 1877: 3, 6). Only the extensive methodological paper on therapy he called Scientific Method and Therapeutic Standpoints" (*Die naturwissenschaftliche Methode und die Standpunkte in der Therapie*), which had a different programmatic relevance (Virchow 1849, see also 1958: 40–66).

As Phillips shows, the use of *"naturwissenschaftlich"* was innocuous until about the 1830s, simply designating "something that had to do with knowledge about nature" (2012: 231). Accordingly, *"wissenschaftlich"* or "scientific" had the broader meaning of designating sound reasoning. But by mid-century, *"naturwissenschaftlich"* began to signify the particularity of the epistemology and method of the natural sciences, as opposed to the human sciences, and was used in a political fashion to separate the two camps ideologically. In other words, the designation *"naturwissenschaftlich"* pointed to the programs by Henle, Wunderlich and others from which Virchow distinguished his concept of scientific medicine in the 1840s and 1850s (they defined their programs as "exact sciences", as can be recalled). That Virchow did not call his program *"naturwissenschaftliche Medicin"*, although he was making clear references to the method of the natural sciences in more than ten occasions of the small sample of texts, which I am discussing here, was because he was drawing a polemical demarcation between his and the physiological programs. He was referring to an idea of scientific methodology as sound and rigorous reasoning, which he had inherited from his teacher Johannes Müller.

My thesis is that Virchow employed the title *"wissenschaftliche Medicin"* (instead of *"naturwissenschaftliche Medicin"*) as a nod to Müller to emphasize this point. Müller had used the term "scientific" still in its broader, harmless meaning, when he, after his appointment to the University of Berlin, began editing a journal in 1834, calling it the *Archiv für Anatomie, Physiologie und wissenschaftliche Medicin.*[57] Müller's position in the history of science and medicine is ambiguous, because as a representative of the first generation of beneficiaries of the new scientific discipline of medicine he is regarded as still a strong proponent of its Romantic inaugurators and of their philosophical interests (Lenoir 1997: 103f.). Despite differences in epistemologies (Virchow was highly critical of Romantic ideals, as I have demonstrated), I want to suggest, however, that Müller and Virchow were connected by sharing a similar institutional or disciplinary condition. Müller was simultaneously appointed to the medical and the philosophi-

---

57 Müller's journal stands in a tradition of scientific publishing that reaches back to Reil's *Archiv für Physiologie* established in 1796 (Lohff 1981: 33).

cal faculty as professor of physiology and anatomy (Lenoir 1997: 104). Virchow, as I already mentioned, was appointed to both the university and the Charité hospital. Müller oversaw an ill-defined academic discipline of "physiology". Though he saw himself primarily as an anatomist, his work spanned studies in human anatomy, animal physiology as well as medical science. The ambiguous constitution of his home discipline required that he create an overarching element around which his heterogeneous work could coalesce and be identified as belonging to a unified scientific discipline – for Müller this was the sound reasoning associated with the methodology of the natural sciences. Virchow's situation was similar in that he needed a way to overarchingly integrate the institution of the laboratory and the clinic as elements of the discipline of medical science. For this purpose, he took inspiration from Müller's strategy.

Müller was known for offering readers of his journal annual critical reviews of the published research conducted in his heterogeneous field. But he did not use it to expound a clear ideological program. Instead, these reviews contain Müller's practical understanding of scientific research. It was mostly contained within his critiques of how others in the field have pursued their work (Lohff 1981: 40–45). Nevertheless, in the first of his annual reviews, Müller was clear that applying "the exact method in empirical analysis of facts is the indispensable task of the natural researcher [*Naturforscher*]." Furthermore, the devising of hypotheses "should only have worth as an incentive for new empirical investigation; and one has to always remember that not the mere erecting of a theory but only the decision about its validity is the actual field of the empirical natural researcher" (Müller 1834: 2f.). In Virchow's words, it sounds like this: "Hypothesis is thus an essential part of scientific investigation, for it represents the thinking that must precede every rational action. [...] The hypotheses and analogies in themselves have no value in scientific investigation except to the extent that they function as entering wedges for further investigation" (Virchow 1958: 33 [Virchow 1847: 12]).

Virchow adopted Müller's idea of scientific rigor and methodology and made it the overarching principle to integrate the different laboratory and clinical approaches into his concept of scientific medicine. Emphasizing its practical instead of its ideological side, Virchow saw that the method of the natural sciences would enable the introduction of what he called an "empirical standpoint" into scientific medicine. Applying it to medical practice allowed to scientifically assess the actions of clinical medicine, instead of, as the "so-called 'physiological school' of therapists" presupposed, only giving theoretical explanations of their therapies (Virchow 1958: 52

[Virchow 1849: 17]). In his text on the natural scientific method and therapy, Virchow therefore made a programmatic statement about what was actually required to work scientifically:

"The scientific method [*naturwissenschaftliche Methode*] [...] enables posing *scientific questions* [*naturwissenschaftliche Fragestellung*]. Everyone capable of properly posing such a question is a natural researcher [*Naturforscher*]. A scientific question is a logical hypothesis based on a known law, which moves forward with the aid of induction and analogy. *Experiment*, itself implicit in the question, gives the answer. [...] Anyone who knows the facts and is capable of logical thought can compel Nature to answer an experimental question, provided that he [sic] has the *materials* necessary for performing the experiment. Natural research [*Naturforschung*] thus presupposes knowledge of the facts, logical thinking, and the appropriate materials" (Virchow 1958: 43f. [1849: 7f.], translation modified).

Consequently, the presupposition for actors of scientific medicine was not their allegiance to the physiological laboratory, but the mere ability to understand and employ the cornerstones of scientific research. Though his emphasis was on microscopy and cellular pathology, Virchow's concept nevertheless depended on a combination of practical and scientific approaches, held together by sound reasoning and pragmatic methodology. For the academic discipline of medicine this meant that medical science became open to research questions and subjects that transcended questions posed in experimental physiology or through physiological measurements. At the same time, making therapy the proper domain of scientific inquiry also altered the expectations associated with medical science: Just as scientific discoveries generally were seen to lay "the ultimate cornerstones for technical progress" (Schauuz/Lax 2018: 68), the promise in medicine now was that more and improved medical research would lead to progress in medical care, i.e., a foundation to tackle all forms and manifestations of sickness in the future with the right clinical means. This is why he believed that progress in science would lead to improvements in public health.

In 1877, Virchow remarked that it was no longer required "to write that scientific medicine is also the best foundation for medical practice" (1958: 149 [Virchow 1877: 9]). Its influence had become self-evident in a variety of practices in the system of academic medicine throughout the German Empire. The program of scientific medicine, as Virchow proposed it, adapted to the ideals of the emerging industrial state of Prussia. It took its bearings from the needs of the working class and also introduced a modern theory of scientific labor into medical science and clinical medicine. His concept furthermore recategorized the relationships within the academic discipline of medicine: as an applied science, medicine hinged on the theoretical foundations and empirical qualifications laid out by pathological physiology. As the name indicated, this science remained indebted to the physiological tradition of Müller, but it no longer functioned to ground medical practice in the way the physiologists proposed (via the epistemic and moral qualities of the scientific doctor trained in measuring bodily processes). As the foundational science for clinical medicine, scientific medicine prescribed a new – and decidedly modern – organization of practical medical knowledge, which outstripped that of its physiological peers, by providing a program to scientifically test and validate medical interventions in a combination of laboratory and clinical observation.

5. The Laboratory and the Making of Clinical Science during the Progressive Era – Scientific Medicine in the USA

The idea of scientific medicine took on a very different form in the North American context than it did in Germany. In this chapter I explain that, rather than constituting the program of an individual actor (like in Germany), US scientific medicine was driven by the aim to reshape the academic system. Between the late-nineteenth and the early-twentieth century, medical education in the USA underwent a significant transition. Aspiring doctors were mostly taught in unscientific and unacademic medical schools during the period immediately after the Civil War, from 1861 to 1865. These institutions had hardly any clinical and laboratory facilities; the faculty was part-time and composed of practicing physicians, who ran the schools for extra income. Fields such as physiology were taught as theoretical subjects and not as practical sciences; and the few individuals devoted to research did so privately – without any material or structural support from their institutions.[58] At the start of the twentieth century, in contrast, medical schools became university affiliated and the medical course began to stand up to academic standards. It included laboratory and clinical training and a full-time faculty responsible for teaching and research (in the natural sciences and later also in clinical fields).

The import of German academic culture into the United States played a crucial part in this remarkable transformation. But historians of American science point to how actors adapted the model of the German university to the American context in a highly selective and modified manner (Benson 1991: 60ff., Bonner 1990, 1995b: 292ff., Ludmerer 1996: 93f., see also Mattingly 2017: 255ff.). At any rate, American physicians had flocked to European medical centers throughout the nineteenth century to receive additional training in areas that schools in North America were unable to provide. They travelled across the Atlantic in the early decades, mainly to acquire expertise in clinical techniques and sciences, especially

---

58 Nevertheless, as John Harley Warner observes, "Medicine was widely acknowledged to be the best occupational choice for a man [sic] who wanted to pursue science in a society that afforded few opportunities to take it up as a profession, and physicians as a group were prominent among the cultivators of science." (1992: 128)

to Paris and Vienna. From the 1860s onward, they increasingly went to German cities to gather practical experiences in the renowned university laboratories (Harvey 1981: 3–30, Warner 1992, Weisz 2006: 72ff.). Some of the physicians who went to the German Empire in the latter part of the century adopted ideals that characterized the science of medicine in the country. They consequently returned as research-minded academics with a "scientific ideology" and views on medical education that "owed much to the example of the German university" (Bonner 1990: 18, see also Maulitz 1979: 92). They now formed the elite of scientists and university administrators that subsequently campaigned to establish features of that research system in US institutions of medical education.

The concept of "scientific medicine" began to emerge as a dominant category in academic and medical discourses in the period in which American physicians were returning from their stays at German universities. It thus is tempting to understand the vocabulary as merely a part of the cultural import. But just as it is too simple to assume that, prior to World War I, US scientists and engineers, for lack of original concepts of science or research, "merely adopted European semantics" (Kaldewey/Schauz 2018: 105), it would also be precipitous to regard the term only as an English-language rendering of the German version. Even though important inspirations were coming from academic medicine in Germany, the cultural understanding of scientific medicine in the United States and its German equivalent varied considerably:

First, in Germany, as I showed, scientific medicine proceeded as a movement within medical academia, whereas in the USA it was a movement to, first, create genuine academic medical institutions. The German term signaled an episode of cultural conflict over the established elite's proper definition of medicine; the American medical elite, in contrast, employed the category with the aim of establishing their scientific interests as an institutional reality in their home country. Therefore, second, while the German term *wissenschaftliche Medicin* connoted the specific program of medicine as an applied science (founded on the independent science of pathology), scientific medicine in the United States functioned more in the sense of Harris's supercategory: It incorporated a broad array of activities and subfields, ranging from pure to applied sciences across to clinical investigation. This more general meaning of "scientific medicine" formed the background to Anglo-American social historians' retroactive portrayals of German academic medicine, although, arguably, it was primarily meant as a program that distinguished itself from the prevailing pure science programs of physiology. They have thereby applied it to include such opposing programs as Wunderlich's and his allies' physiological medicine and Virchow's program (e.g., Lenoir 1997, Tuchman 1993). Crucially, though, while scientific medicine had one clearly defined meaning in the German university, its counterpart in the Unites States, as I demonstrate below, harbored two largely distinct notions, namely, (1) that of the "basic" medical laboratory sciences and (2) that of clinical science.

The American medical profession saw two separate disciplines emerge under the name of scientific medicine at the end of the nineteenth and the start of the twentieth century. Scholars have thoroughly investigated how the American medical elite inspired by the German university and its medical training campaigned to have their ideals of science and laboratory investigation installed into the domestic system (Bonner 1990, 1995b, Fye 1987, Ludmerer 1996, see also Kohler 1982: 121–157). Hence, I here concentrate on how, in comparison, the idea of *clinical science* was defined, and on how its disciplinary identity was institutionalized in the USA. From a diachronic perspective, this model is still visible as the clinical culture in much of the Western hemisphere, i.e., in the large research hospitals that harbor facilities for treating patients and performing medical research (Keating/Cambrosio 2003).

Semantic evidence for this disciplinary differentiation can be drawn from the appearance of the term "preclinical" with the prefix "pre" in the 1910s, used to designate the laboratory sciences in contradistinction to clinical science. The label indicated, in the words of Lewellys Barker, physician-in-chief at Johns Hopkins, that "the time has passed when the work of the clinics could be regarded as something that is not scientific – as something merely practical or technical to be sharply distinguished from the 'theoretical' or 'scientific' work of the preclinical sciences" (1916: 632). The notions of preclinical and clinical science nevertheless overlapped in their core scientific values, as I will show. With the words of Becher and Trowler, I claim that they were of the same tribe, but that they settled on different territories, that is, they differed in their conception and orientation. Preclinical and clinical sciences shared the ideal of the scientific method, although in the American academic discourse this meant something different than in the vocabulary employed in Germany. The aim in the United States was to create a new clinical science that adhered to the experimental ideals of the laboratory. Ultimately, this new science was founded on a new institution. As such, clinical science could now be performed through inputs from their own clinical laboratories, which had acquired important administrative and service functions in large hospitals by 1920. "The main function of these laboratories", as Kohler notes, "was to provide routine laboratory tests for diagnosis or therapy, but the professional staffs were also expected to cooperate with the clinical staffs, to instruct interns and medical students in advanced analytical procedures and to do research" (1982: 231).

How can it be explained that, unlike in Germany, where the category *scientific medicine* entailed the integration of the clinic and lab, scientific medicine in the US context meant the formation of an independent discipline of clinical science next to the medical laboratory sciences? The general answer is that the ideals of science had to be accommodated to the dominant orientation on practice that characterized medicine and society in the nineteenth-century United States. American physicians "agreed that practice, not the possession of or access to special knowledge, was in the final analysis the source of the medical practitioner's authority and identity" (Warner 1992: 125, see also Warner 1986). Consequently, arguments for founding medicine on science needed a legitimation that pointed to its usefulness for practical medicine, while in Germany, in contrast, medicine was defined in terms of knowledge basis and academic credentials. Though the German medical elite was split internally over questions of whether the proper scientific basis for medicine should derive from laws of organic nature explored in laboratories or from the practical experience physicians collected through empirical observation in the clinics, they did not call into question the academic status of medicine. University affiliation provided German medicine with authority, whereas the situation in the US proved to be more complicated.

Historians of American medicine warn their readers about the need to be careful not to understand the profession as too monolithic when looking at scientific medicine in the US (Ludmerer 1996: 118f., Warner 1995: 178f., see also Weisz 2006: 74f.). Different to Germany, the academic physician and the ordinary practitioner here belonged to different communities. "The clinical professor in Germany was primarily an academic man," Bonner observes, "whereas the American teacher-practitioner was firmly rooted among the patients in the home soil of the city where he lived" (Bonner 1995b: 284, see also Harvey 1981: 133). Consequently, the academic doctor and the routine practitioner had different reasons for adopting the ideals of scientific medicine: first-row advocates "saw the greater infusion of experimental science into American medicine as a vehicle for scientific career making" and progressive medical practitioners viewed science "as a vehicle for augmenting cultural authority and income" (Warner 1995: 179).

The strategy of academic actors in the US to institutionalize the medical laboratory sciences as a primary form of occupation superficially resembled that of their German counterparts. It involved advocating for the methods of the natural sciences as a requirement for medical training. But whereas German actors claimed that training in the scientific method enabled doctors to behave like a scientist at the bedside, the reasoning in the Progressive Era differed slightly but significantly. The argument was that training in the methods of the natural sciences was appropriate for both the scientist *and* physician, because essentially the practice of science and clinical medicine were the same, just applied to different objects (Flexner 1910). In the last decade of the nineteenth century, it was accepted that the concept of scientific medicine entailed the idea of practical medicine as an applied science based on the laboratory sciences (this, in a sense, resembles the false friend understanding, which I mentioned in the previous chapter [Davis 1891, see also Warner 1991, 1986: 235–283]). Not even two decades later, however, actors called for a "pure science" of clinical medicine, that is, for basing clinical medicine on an independent institution of clinical science, distinguished from the pure laboratory sciences on the one side and the obligations of medical practice on the other (Meltzer 1909, see also Harvey 1981: 112–126). Clinical scientists shared the values of pure science. But instead of aiming at furthering the theoretical (biological) knowledge of medicine, like their counterparts in Germany, they strove to improve medical practice with the aid of modern science. As a result, while scientific medicine in Germany was just one name among several, the American equivalent was more encompassing since it entailed the institutionalization of science for the equal furthering of both medical theory and clinical practice.

In the following, I will reconstruct how the category of scientific medicine in the US absorbed the medical profession's existing structural preferences for practice and together with the ideals imported from Germany transformed them into two distinct disciplinary identities of academic medicine. I want to argue that the separation into different institutions, due to their different orientations to practice and science, also prepared the later transformation of medical science into biomedicine. Adopting central concepts of German laboratory science to the medical discourse of the Progressive Era made them lose most of their restrictive and elitist German undertones. Consequently, these concepts provided more of a general framework of values in which the laboratory sciences and the clinical science of American scientific medicine were able to develop their individual cultural characteristics and identities. At the same time, however, the two scientific cultures arrived at somewhat crossed relations with each other. Different from Germany, where scientific medicine meant an applied science that maintained connections to the clinic, the establishment of independent clinical laboratories as auxiliaries to clinical science paradoxically caused the conceptual separation of the institution of the clinic from that of the medical laboratory sciences.[59] As a consequence, this left the latter sciences with merely a rhetorical link to clinical medicine. From this point, these sciences have been devoted to research issues that became increasingly indistinguishable in their biological and/or medical trajectories. As I demonstrate in the next chapter, institutions nominally "medical", such as university medical schools or the National Institutes of Health, became entrusted with furthering research that factually belonged to the basic biological sciences. By the end of World War II, this led to an ambiguous situation of research jurisdiction and of funding in biology and medicine, necessitating a new categorization (Appel 2000). The basis for this unclear situation, which is addressed later in this chapter, derived from the inability to define academic biology in the US before the twentieth century and the resulting imbrication of biological and medical cultures.

I. German Ideals of Academic Medicine in the American Discourse

To understand how the disciplinary structures of biomedicine were prearranged in the making of academic medicine, I unfurl the emergence of the idea of scientific medicine in the US. How did it come to comprise two independent medical disciplines – that of clinical science and the preclinical sciences? These two evolved in succession, not in parallel, which is owed to the fact that the scientific ideals of the medical laboratory, in a sense, subsequently began to rub off onto practically oriented actors through their education in the new methods. To make sense of this development, I trace how medical actors inspired by German science introduced academic ideals, like the "commitment to the full-time system, the experimental method, and the research ethic" (Fye 1987: 207), into the American discourse. Nevertheless, I will highlight how they were transformed into having a specifically North American meaning.

---

59 Such a separation was, of course, not absolute since clinical science continued to draw on laboratory practices and knowledge. But the emergence of clinical laboratories was also accompanied by the development of a culture specific to these places and distinct from that of the medical research laboratory (Kohler 1981: 237–243, Reiser 1979: 139ff.).

Bonner analyzed how the didactic ideals that American physicians brought back from their visits to Germany differed from the original, although they tirelessly "proselytized the strengths of the German system" – high overall standards, the pursuit of original research work, academic freedom, the "unity of research and teaching", highly specialized fields and the appropriate research facilities headed by prestigious scientists (1990: 19, see also Bonner 1995a: 292ff.). At the same time, however, American reformers withheld important aspects that defined medical education at German universities. They regarded them as undesirable or unsuitable for the American context, "notably the research-oriented institute, the private teacher or *dozent*, the great power of the professor, and the freedom of students to select their own courses" (Bonner 1995a: 292). Academic medicine in Germany was characterized by a two-tier system. The great mass of undergraduates was only minimally exposed to the workings of the laboratory or the clinic, while advanced students received personal laboratory experience and facetime with professors.[60] "Lectures", therefore, as Bonner notes, "remained a principal and dominant medium of teaching medicine [in Germany]" (1990: 20). Accordingly, a clear separation of laboratory research and advanced training "from undergraduate teaching in crowded lecture halls, clinics, and laboratories" existed (ibid: 30). The medical education that was established in the US, in contrast, was infused with democratic or egalitarian values, making "a good medical education" the standard for all students, "in contrast to Europe, where the best training was reserved for the elite" (Ludmerer 1996: 94, see also Bonner 1990: 31). Clinical experience, for example, played a greater role in the education of physicians in the US after 1870 than it did in Germany. More importantly, though, in the medical institutions that the American elite intended for their home country, undergraduate students also received the kind of extensive laboratory training reserved only for advanced students in nineteenth-century Germany. According to Bonner, the "fragile university medical schools of the late nineteenth century" in the US did not allow to distinguish between "normal teaching and advanced work" (1990: 26).

This difference in national style can be explained with the high regard for praxis that prevailed in the medical world of the US (Warner 1986). While German professors could allow themselves to introduce scientific ideals into medical training to further the academic quality of medical students, their American peers needed to dress these ideals up as improve-

---

60 I noted in the previous chapter that eminent scientists like Hermann von Helmholtz refrained from their duties in medical education.

ments of graduates' practical proficiencies. Consequently, one key concept of medical education in Germany – the scientific method – acquired a meaning mostly devoid of its more restrictive and elitist connotations in the New World. In Germany, as argued above, ideology drew a clear line between the laboratory and the clinic. Apart from protagonists like Virchow, who employed the idea of scientific methodology with a practical aim in mind, German scientists introduced the scientific method as a pedagogical ideal primarily to foster recruitment into medical research.

No such ideological distinction between clinical and preclinical sciences existed in the US Here, more generally, rationales to justify the pure science ideal "gradually shifted [...] towards utilitarian arguments" (Kaldewey/Schauz 2018: 115). In medicine specifically, it required adapting the idea of the scientific method to a practically oriented climate and framing it straightforwardly as a means to improve medical care. The employed strategy accordingly dropped the categorical distinction between work done in the laboratory and in the clinic. To illustrate in detail how the strategy of equating the mental capacities of the researcher and those of the medical practitioner worked, I refer to the single most important document associated with medical reform in the US – the Carnegie Foundation's Bulletin Number Four, *Medical Education in the United States and Canada*, compiled by the educational reformer Abraham Flexner and published in 1910.

The so-called Flexner Report is a scathing critique of the system of American medical education at the turn of the century. The report is reminiscent of the muckraking literature that was popular during the Progressive Era, in which authors exposed the corruption inherent in established institutions of American society. Abraham Flexner visited all medical schools in the US and Canada to examine their entrance requirements, training of the faculty and quality teaching facilities, financial resources and access to hospitals. The inquiry had damning results (Flexner 1910: 27–51). Of the over one hundred and fifty existing schools, he recommended that the vast majority ought to be shut down due to their poor quality. He saw that that they were graduating a too large number of doctors of a far too disparate quality. Only a few schools could in his opinion boast the appropriate academic standards – for which the Johns Hopkins Medical School, opened in 1893, stood as the shining example (Flexner 1910: 12). Flexner was an advocate of removing medical education from the control of practitioners and placing it under the surveillance of the university system. He designed a four-year medical curriculum as a model for this purpose, divided equally between training in the preclinical and clinical sciences, complete with the requirement of full-time faculty in both fields, which illustrated his educational ideal.

The history, context and implications of the Flexner Report for medicine haven been thoroughly researched and it is beyond the scope of my book to recite these works here (see e.g., Berliner 1985, Ludmerer 1996: 166–190, Mattingly 2017: 218f. McClelland 2013, Wheatley 1989). Generally, the text can be said to be a public document that is rare in having "had such a deep impact on any cultural activity" in the US and around the globe (McClelland 2013). It is interesting for my argument precisely because of what historian of medicine Kenneth Ludmerer called its "galvanizing effect on public sentiment" (1996: 167). It acts as an example of the accepted language and concepts to talk and write about science and medicine, propagated by the elite of academic physicians since the 1870s. The report uses the term "scientific medicine" only sporadically but definingly (Flexner 1910: 9, 53, 157, 158, 162). This may indicate that the term had become a common category in the academic discourse at the time of the report's publication and had little need for explication.[61] According to Ludmerer, the term scientific medicine meant two things for Flexner: first of all, it meant the acceptance of physics, chemistry and biology as "the intellectual foundation of modern medicine" (1996: 174). Secondly, it was the realization of the "scientific method applied to practice as well as research" (ibid.).

Flexner gives a lengthy elaboration of why the method underlying sciences like physics, chemistry or biology is "just as applicable to practice as to research" (1910: 53). According to Ludmerer, "Flexner abhorred the 'rule-of-thumb' practitioner", who oriented his/her[62] actions according to protocol and not by his/her own critical thought (1996: 175). Like proponents of the pure science ideal, who viewed the products of science as a foundation for the practical application of knowledge in engineering and other areas (Kaldewey/Schauz 2018: 117), Flexner thus saw that science would help structure the practical aspects of medicine. He accordingly explained that, at the basis, the professional actions of the researcher and

---

61 The report, furthermore, refers to "pre-medical" instead of 'preclinical' "sciences", "work", or "courses" (Flexner 1910: 30, 33, 43, 47, 71, 77, 78, 83, 210, 211, 212).

62 Although women were not formally restricted from medical education, and medical schools specifically for women were established in the nineteenth century, the existing cultural climate in many places of the United States nevertheless still prohibited that women receive academic medical training.

the medical practitioner were essentially the same and could be structured using the scientific method:

> "And just as it makes no difference to science whether usable data be obtained from a slide beneath a microscope or from a sick man stretched out on a cot, so the precise nature of the act or experiment is immaterial: it matters not in the slightest, from the standpoint of scientific logic, whether the step take the form of administering a dose of calomel, operating for appendicitis, or stimulating a particular convolution of a frog's brain with an electric current. The logical position is in all three cases identical" (Flexner 1910: 92).

Flexner argued at length that both scientist and doctor work with theories or hypotheses, which is in the case of medical practice "called a diagnosis"; that both are "confronted with a definite situation", which the scientist observes for "taking all the facts", whereas for the physician the "patient's history, conditions, symptoms, form his data"; for both, this "suggests a line of action" (Flexner ibid: 55). And just in the way that the researcher's mind "flies like a shuttle" between theory and fact, allowing him to "understand, relate, and control phenomena", so the competency of the medical practitioner is determined by the "ability to heed the response which nature thus makes to his ministrations" (ibid.). Flexner is tireless to repeat that the "practicing physician and the 'theoretical' scientist are thus engaged in doing the same sort of thing" (ibid: 92); "They employ the same method, the same sort of intelligence" (ibid: 56); "Investigation and practice are thus one in spirit, method, and object" (ibid.); "The progress of science and the scientific or intelligent practice of medicine employ, therefore, exactly the same technique" (ibid: 55, see also Weisz 2006: 128).[63]

The dogmatic insistence on the sameness of the intellectual properties grounding the scientist's and physician's actions is, of course, an exaggeration. Experiment serves as a pedagogical tool in medical training through which the physician's "powers of observation" are fostered to allow a perception of disease in adequate detail (ibid.). "In each a supposition, – whether expressed or implied, whether called theory or diagnosis, – based on supposedly adequate observation, submits itself to the test of an

---

63 Flexner does, however, concede that if "we differentiate investigator and practitioner, it is because in the former case action is leisurely and indirect, in the latter case, immediate and anxious." Nevertheless, "the mental qualities involved are the same." (1910: 56)

experiment" (ibid: 92). But it is questionable whether it is really flattering to the practicing physician to have his/her actions compared to that of an experiment. From a sociological perspective, important structural differences underlie the actions of modern scientists and physicians. While the one, for example, downright embraces uncertainty, the other risks losing his/her professional authority over its disclosure in the interaction with a patient. In other words, while the open communication of still uncertain knowledge is a central feature of scientific practice and progress, the medical practitioner must necessarily conceal the uncertainty underlying his/her actions, and compensate it with subjective factors, to maintain the trust of his/her patient (Stichweh 1994a: 296f.). The fact downplayed by Flexner is that in the "twilight region" between knowledge and uncertainty about the nature of disease "the physician may indeed only surmise", although he is fully aware of the fact of only surmising (ibid: 55). This is, however, one of the crucial factors constituting the difference between science and a practical profession – one that differentiates experiment and the operations of diagnosis and therapy.

Be that as it may, in the American context, "with its emphasis on the clinical branches at the expense of the scientific subjects" (Fye 1987: 107), eliminating the conceptual boundary between the actions of the scientific and practical professions in medicine was required in order to justify the large-scale establishment of facilities for research and training in science. These were foundational for institutional arrangements that would ensure recruitment of students endowed with the proper cultural repertoire into the new occupation of medical science. The removal of the conceptual difference between scientific and medical practice has also contributed to the bias evident in sociological and historical literature today. Conflating the idea of both practices resulted in the creation of an identity for medicine as a professional practice, which is at the same time scientific, instead of viewing it as a profession next to that of a scientific discipline.

The underlying rationale employed by medical actors in the US towards the end of the nineteenth century was similar to that used by their German counterparts more than two generations earlier: only a direct exposure to the phenomena of nature, rather than relaying them through lectures or textbooks, would allow the student to develop the mental qualities necessary to pursue either a scientific or practical profession in medicine (Bonner 1995a: 236ff.). "What helps" the student of medicine, according to Barker, "is less the facts which he learns, or the memory of the experiments he makes, than the establishment in him of the conception that in order really to understand it is necessary to come into direct personal contact with the object to be understood" (1908: 607, see also Flexner 1910: 53). Like the German reformers, they stressed that working with the methods of scientific investigation in the laboratory would provide a training of the senses unmatched by mere recitation (Harvey 1981: 34, Ludmerer 1996: 65).

There was a slight but crucial difference between the two national cultures, however. The German argument read that such a training would primarily foster intellectual and moral capabilities from which appropriate instructions for action could then derive naturally. It was directed at the academic who, as a well and comprehensively educated person, would automatically know how to act. The American idea, in turn, was more pragmatic in the literal sense; in that the priority for action was the reason for acquiring the theoretical equipment since it taught one how to approach a problem practically. Ludmerer accordingly argues that the concept of "progressive education" of the early elite of medical scientists in the US was identical to that popularized by the philosopher John Dewey at the start of the twentieth century and interlaced into Flexner's report (1996: 63–71, 176, see also Flexner 1910: 68 n.2).

The egalitarian understanding at the heart of the scientific method in the US did not only eliminate the strict boundary between the scientific and practical occupations of medicine, but it also linked the concept of scientific medicine to the idea of social progress characteristic of pragmatism. For Dewey, just as for the actors in medical science, the prevailing ideology was that the same "scientific habit of mind" or "scientific habit of thought" applied to not only the activity of research, but to virtually all circumstances of modern everyday life – including patient care (Dewey 1910: 126, Barker 1908: 607, Flexner 1910: 157, see also Ludmerer 1996: 67). In a lecture given to the American Association for the Advancement of Science at the start of the twentieth century, Dewey explained that science was not defined by its subject matter, but that it rather constituted "a mode of intelligent practice, an [sic] habitual disposition of mind" (ibid: 125). Its value lay therefore less in its content but in its procedures, in "the knowledge of the ways by which anything is entitled to be called knowledge" (ibid.). Knowledge of the methods of scientific inquiry were accordingly more than just the benchmark of a small scientific elite:

> "Scientific method is not just a method which it has been found profitable to pursue in this or that abstruse subject for purely technical reasons. It represents the only method of thinking that has proved fruitful in any subject – that is what we mean when we call it scientific. It is not a peculiar development of thinking for highly specialized ends; it

is thinking so far as thought has become conscious of its proper ends and of the equipment indispensable for success in their pursuit" (ibid: 127).

The crucial aspect of scientific thinking, which a training in the method enabled, was for Dewey therefore the cultivation of a critical disposition in the mind of the modern individual. Science and its method were not only for "highly specialized ends" – this also meant that it represented a way of thinking equally applicable to medical matters. In his book *How We Think*, published in 1910, he contrasts the scientific method with what he calls the empirical method. The latter is characterized by the construction of general facts from the indiscriminate association of observations with each other. It thus enforces established customs and beliefs through the perception of ostensibly similar cases (Dewey 1997: 145–149). Thinking scientifically with the aid of the scientific method, in contrast, allows for innovation in knowledge and behavior to occur, because of its change in attitude from the simple dependence on "routine and custom" to the "intelligent regulation of existing conditions". While the empirical method is characterized by passivity, since it must rely on cases being presented to the individual to be realized, science employs the experimental method, which is characterized by the ability to actively vary the conditions of observation (ibid: 151). "The empirical method inevitably magnifies the influences of the past; the experimental method throws into relief the possibilities of the future" (ibid: 154). The use of the scientific method as an ideal for medical training in the US, therefore, did not only imply a more democratic understanding of academic medicine compared to Germany, but it also infused ideals of science into the institutions of laboratory and clinical research, amongst which progressing the scientific knowledge of medicine was a central goal.

II. From Applied Science to the Pure Science of Clinical Medicine

The conceptual shift from medical practice as an applied science of the laboratory to being founded on the independent discipline of clinical science is an example of the institutional ramifications of the Progressive Era understanding of medical education in the United States. The idea of medicine as an applied science, as pointed out, developed in Germany as the result of basing medicine on the method of the natural sciences laboratory as opposed to the rigorous empiricism of clinical medicine. According to historian of medicine John Harley Warner, the development of a program of "applied medical science" in the US also resulted from efforts to oppose the empirical approach to clinical practice (1991: 461, see also Warner 1986: 247ff.). The crucial difference, however, was that in Germany the conflict between the scientific ideals of the laboratory and the empiricism of the clinic was about defining the proper basis of academic medicine. In the US, in contrast, it revolved around establishing the basis for professional practice, namely, a "science of therapeutics" for medical practitioners (Warner 1986: 247). The "science" of empiricism ruled in American medicine from the early decades of the nineteenth century to the end of the Civil War. Physicians trained in Europe had imported it especially from the Clinical School tradition of the Paris hospitals. After the 1860s, the approach was deemed unable to support a truly scientific basis for therapeutics.[64] At this point, instead, "making therapeutics more rational by basing it on laboratory experimentation meant making it more scientific" (ibid: 248).

In 1891, the eminent physician and charter member of the American Medical Association, Nathan Smith Davis, gave a lecture in Chicago titled "The Basis of Scientific Medicine and the Proper Methods of Investigation". The talk was an indication of the successful introduction of the laboratory sciences into medicine in the US. However, it still referred to the dominance of the medical laboratory for practice and did not yet imply the idea of a separate clinical science. Although his conception of scientific medicine differs somewhat from the movement of "physiological therapeutics", which Warner describes as part of American medicine in the second half of the nineteenth century (1984: 235–257, see also Warner 1991), the core rationale of both was very similar. Davis remarked only the need to substitute "the word *pathology* for physiology", arguing that "Therapeutics relates to the application of remedies for the control, not of healthy or physiological processes, but of morbid or pathological condi-

---

64 The Paris Clinical School at the end of the eighteenth century has entered the annals of medicine for relating empirical observations in the clinic with insights from dissections at the end of the eighteenth century. Michel Foucault (1976) has famously suggested that this resulted in a general change in medical epistemology. The main argument is that the systematic use of clinical observation, including physical methods of diagnosis, and the practice of pathological anatomy henceforth enabled physicians to "see" disease and how it was located inside the patient's body. This moved the idea of sickness from premodern understandings and abstract ideas to a concept of disease that centered on disturbances in the human body itself, like anatomical lesions.

tions, and is consequently applied pathology" (1891: 115).[65] He conceded, however, that physiology was the basis for a science of pathology. Thus, according to Davis' categorization of scientific medicine,

> "the great fields of natural and physical sciences known as anatomy, histology, physiology, pathology, medical chemistry and materia medica, constitute the acknowledged basis of modern medicine; while therapeutics or practical medicine, surgery, and sanitation or preventive medicine, are strictly applied sciences developed by the same methods of observation, experimentation and induction that have brought into existence all other inductive sciences" (ibid.).

It is worth noting that Davis calls medical disciplines "great fields of natural and physical sciences" to make their common heritage and conception unmistakable. However, the "same method" in Davis' remarks did not so much refer to the same education of the scientific and clinical practitioner – this was only slowly starting to become an established fact among the academic medical elite at the time of Davis' lecture (Fye 1987: 206ff.). Instead, it referred to the use of the same procedures and techniques – and implied even the same facilities – to investigate both the basis of modern medicine and ways to improve clinical practice. Davis was very much in line with the physiological protagonists of mid-nineteenth-century Germany. The practitioner was to receive an exact orientation on how to treat a patient via study of normal and abnormal phenomena and of the effects of drugs in the laboratory (Warner 1986: 250f.). "Therapeutics was to be advanced", Warner notes, "by reasoning from the laboratory to the bedside" (ibid: 246). A common comparison used to emphasize the relation between laboratory science and clinical action, therefore, was that between mathematics and engineering, "implying that the reasoning called for in the treatment of disease was mechanical and almost automatic" (Warner 1991: 458, see also Davis 1891: 115). It was meant to emphasize an ideal of exactness and precision that would supposedly characterize therapeutics based on the ideals and finding of the laboratory sciences.

From the early twentieth century onward, it no longer sufficed for clinicians in the US to apply the knowledge of the medical science departments to practical medicine. In 1909, at the first meeting of the new Association

---

65 The semblance with Virchow's program seems striking. But it needs to be remembered that his program entailed the integration of clinic and laboratory as equals. Davis, as will become obvious, was implying more the sort of reasoning characteristic of the program of physiological medicine in Germany.

for Clinical Research, for example, physician and physiologist Samuel Meltzer advocated for establishing clinical medicine as a genuine and autonomous science. Four years later, in 1913, the physician-in-chief at Johns Hopkins was calling for establishing the according facilities for such a science – namely, research laboratories adjacent to clinics in hospitals. Germany witnessed similar ambitions toward the end of the nineteenth century. But here clinical medicine was construed in demarcation from the laboratory sciences. With the takeover of the medical curriculum by the natural sciences, clinicians had (again) begun to react with criticism toward the close of the nineteenth century (Bonner 1995a: 269–274, see also Bleker 1987/88). The techniques of the laboratory (especially in the wake of bacteriology) increasingly allowed a sole reliance on animal experiment for studying disease, causing a separation of medical science from the clinical object of study, i.e., the human subject. Clinical researchers-teachers, in turn, felt threatened in their professional identity and reemphasized the importance of practical clinical experience for medical students. According to historian Russell Maulitz, in this context, "German physicians seized on two basic tools": on the one hand, they revived the nosographical tradition of their predecessors, "the classification and description of disease in the older, natural-historical mode"; on the other, clinicians reacted with "their own technological innovations", with bed-side methods "to permit observation of previously unexplored body orifices" (1979: 95). Similar to developments earlier in the century, German clinical medicine thus defined itself methodologically in contradistinction to the method of the laboratory sciences. The establishment of laboratories in clinical institutes therefore merely meant that the natural sciences were serving as auxiliaries (Bleker 1987/88: 43).

The category of clinical medicine as a pure science, which Meltzer introduced and Barker indirectly adopted, did not necessarily oppose the idea of practical medicine as an applied science. Instead, it argued for placing clinical practice on an autonomous scientific basis separate from the department of the medical laboratory sciences. In a sense, this move was a direct reference to the idea of scientific medicine introduced by Virchow after the mid-nineteenth century in Germany. It was designed to provide a new institutional basis for practical medicine, just as Virchow had designed a new basis with the science of pathology. "I am of the opinion", Meltzer stated, "that clinical medicine as it exists now is made up of two constituents: one part has all the elements of a pure science and ought to be coordinate to the other pure sciences of medicine, and the other part is the real practice of medicine, an applied science which has many elements of an art" (1909: 508). The concept of "pure science", as it was floated at the turn of the century, employed two contradictory meanings that actors could appropriate. It served as "a distinct activity separate from technology and commerce" or as foundational to the realms of applied science and technology (Kaldewey/Schauz 2018: 115). The main reason to employ the category of pure science here was to argue for the academic status of clinical science and for its institutional independence from practical medicine, since currently the subject was still taught mostly by active physicians "who devote most of their time and energies to their practice and to the golden fruit it bears" (Meltzer 1909: 510).

Barker's reasoning led to the same result, although it pursued a different route. To him, "all the sciences, with the possible exception of mathematics, are largely 'applied sciences'" (1913: 732). Internal medicine, the main province of clinical medicine, "is, of all the biological sciences, the one to which the largest number of other sciences contribute facts for application" (ibid.). Accordingly, he endowed the science of clinical medicine with qualities of a pure science, arguing that even as an applied science it had to grow in its own way and required its own professional actors to do so: "each science is creative and has to devise methods of its own; even when a new fact in a science basal to it is applicable, the application actually has to be made" (ibid.). The point of both Barker and Meltzer was to underline that the growth of medical knowledge coming from the laboratories did not automatically equal a growth in knowledge for practical medicine. Thus, only if clinical medicine was treated as an independent science, equipped with the according features (and not simply as the endpoint of laboratory research), would it advance in a similar fashion to the other medical sciences. "Clinical science will not thrive through chance investigations by friendly neighbors from the adjoining practical and scientific domains", Meltzer argued (1909: 509); and for Barker it was a still common misunderstanding "that the laboratories of the non-clinical sciences can be called upon to do the laboratory work of clinical science" (1913: 735).

Working from a background in which a new generation of physicians had just been extensively trained in the new methods and techniques of the laboratory sciences, the advocates of clinical science in the US did not want to oppose this foundation of medicine. In Germany, scientific medicine and clinical medicine were distinguished methodologically. But in the US the demarcation was drawn less based on the methods applied than on the subjects they were applied to. Physiology and anatomy provided knowledge of normal structures and processes, pathology that of abnormal changes in the body. "To clinical medicine is left", Meltzer accordingly concluded, "the study of the phenomena and their sequence as they occur in a living body during the entire course of a disease" (1909: 508). Observational methods played a key role in defining the practice and research of clinical medicine in Germany, but American clinicians embraced the methods of the experimental laboratory sciences for promoting their cause. Although Meltzer defines "the domain of clinical research" as "the study of the natural history of disease, their physiology and their pharmacology", he brings it in proximity not to the methods characteristic of German clinical medicine but to the "experimental methods" of the "pure sciences" (ibid: 509). It was widely accepted in the American academic discourse at the start of the twentieth century that the methods of the experiment were applicable to the study of disease and therapeutics. Leading research in the fields of internal medicine, paediatrics, surgery and gynaecology was no longer simply understood in terms of describing disease manifestations in the clinic. "Rather, research in these fields, like research in the basic sciences, had become laboratory-based" (Ludmerer 1996: 208f., see also Flexner 1910: 101f.).

The professional qualities and *habitus* of the individuals pursuing research in clinical science, at first sight, thus differed little from those pursuing "pure" lab research. According to Meltzer, they should not simply be trained in "other sciences of medicine" but should in fact have done "investigations in one or more of these pure sciences" to be acquainted with "careful scientific method and imbued with a scientific spirit"; they should "acquire the habitus and the taste of the investigator, the scientist, which may stick with them for life" (1909: 509). They were thus clearly of the same academic tribe as the preclinical scientists. For Barker, the objects of clinical research needed to be "intellectualized partly by accurate training in the most recent clinical technique, partly by the previous education in the methods, facts and hypothesis of the non-clinical sciences" (1913: 734). Most importantly, though, the new clinical scientists, using Becher's and Trowler's terms, occupied a different territory than the preclinical scientists. They had to "select clinical research as the main field of their scientific activity", applying the scientific spirit acquired through medical education to the furthering and cultivation of knowledge specific to the field of clinical science (Meltzer 1909: 509).

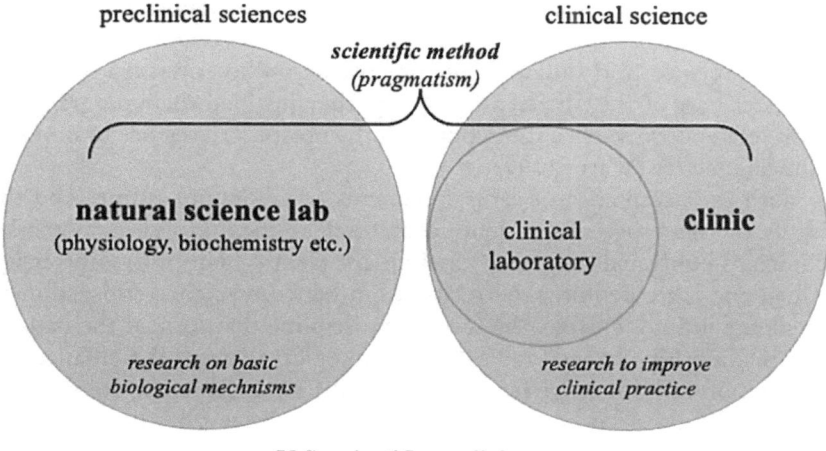

preclinical sciences   clinical science

scientific method
(pragmatism)

natural science lab
(physiology, biochemistry etc.)

clinical
laboratory

clinic

research on basic
biological mechnisms

research to improve
clinical practice

U.S. scientific medicine

Figure 5.1: Schema of the structural relationship between preclinical sciences and clinical science in the US idea of scientific medicine (my depiction).

It is interesting to note that in the hands of the clinicians the scientific method, which constituted an emblem of democracy and progress, turned into a central element of a larger scheme to constitute their own scientific elite. It became applied to genuinely clinical problems outside the reach of the lab researcher. Whereas laboratory scientists in medical departments could study disease *in vitro* or in animals, only clinical scientists could study disease in humans. Physician and medical historian A. McGehee Harvey identified this as the emergence of "a new type of medical worker", stylized as a hybrid actor based on the convictions that clinical science was a genuine science, which devoted itself legitimately to the study of disease, thus bridging "the work of clinic and laboratory, physician and basic scientist" (1981: 116, see also Barker 1913: 735).[66] The idea of the new clinical scientist was, therefore, not simply distinct from that of the German clinical professor, but also from the American medical scientist. It combined the scientific virtues of the laboratory scientist with the general orientation of the practitioner (figure 5.1), so that the new breed of clini-

---

66   I referred to the prototypical creation of this figure in the previous chapter, in Virchow's reframing of the clinic and consequently also of the clinician as a practitioner and researcher. It will become relevant again when we discuss the concept of translational research in chapter 7.

cians "adopted some of the values of the biomedical scientists but not their professional goals" (Kohler 1982: 221). Unlike the laboratory researcher of medical science, and similar to the practitioners who embraced science in the later part of the nineteenth century, they justified their program not with reference to science itself, but with the prospect of science to improve clinical practice (Warner 1991: 461).

With the acceptance of central elements of laboratory culture and the ideals of the progressive scientific method as their professional marks, clinicians cultivated their own disciplinary identity within the university. Albeit the logic defining the relationship between science and action in medicine did not change, the scientific discipline that formed the basis of this relationship changed radically. Physiological therapeutics entailed the application of knowledge from the medical science laboratory to the bedside. In clinical science, it meant applying knowledge from the laboratory of the clinical department or hospital. Consequently, the new clinicians employed similar comparisons with engineering or technology. For engineers, physics provides the methods and ideas from which conceptions for materials and layout are constructed; for clinicians, physiology and pathology provide the basis for conceiving of states of disease and therapies. "It was not simply a matter of applying basic science", Robert Kohler attentively notes, "but of creating new basic applied-science disciplines. Clinical scientists' ultimate purpose was to cure the sick, just as the aim of engineering was to build dams or machines" (1982: 221).

Consequently, with a new discipline wedged between the laboratory sciences and clinical practice, the former became more removed from clinical reality. "Without the development of such a department of clinical science the efficiency of the practice of internal medicine will lag behind, no matter how progressive the allied sciences of medicine are and how great their efforts to be useful to medicine might be" (Meltzer 1909: 510, see also Barker 1913: 736f.). The reference to medicine's "allied sciences", which Meltzer used, as I show in the next chapter, manifests a significant semantic development: with a new knowledge foundation for practical medicine, "pure" medical science began to transition closer to biology and further away from the problems of clinical medicine.

III. Institutional Ambiguities of Medical and Biological Research

The Relation of biology and medicine in the USA at the turn to the twentieth century was ambiguous. It was affected by the conceptual migration of medical science away from the clinic and this development impact the institutional structures of academic medicine and science. To get a better picture of how American academic structures prearranged the idea of biomedicine at the end of the nineteenth and the start of the twentieth century, I want to briefly sketch the development of academic biology at the time. My focus is only on very general institutional developments, not on the different biological schools nor on the contexts of application of biology, which there were many. Academic biology was still an ill-defined entity in the US at the end of the nineteenth century and mainly split between the specialties of zoology and botany (figure 5.2). Historians of science furthermore reveal the "clearly discernible cleavages between the biomedical [sic] sciences, based in medical schools, and those biological sciences primarily based in universities" (Appel 1991: 89, see also Appel 1987, Kohler 1982, Pauly 1984). The reference to location is crucial, as will become obvious, since effectively it was the only factor demarcating the disciplinary cultures of experimental biology and medical science.

Characteristic of biology's development in the late-nineteenth century US, in comparison to medicine, was its fragmentation. While the Flexner report was the manifestation of an interest for centralized standards of academic medicine, biology developed at several centers with different emphases and orientations (Pauly 1984). It was unable to organize itself as a discipline even after the start of the twentieth century (Appel 1991). Kohler notes that American biology at the time still lacked the characteristics of a "homogenous community" and the "unusually authoritative core elite" of other fields. Instead, biology constituted "a congeries of competing and contentious subspecialties or subcultures," which were connected to various fields like medicine, agriculture, psychology or the management of natural resources, "all of which offered attractive but competing opportunities for discipline building" (Kohler 1991: 108, see also Appel 1991).

The reforming medical schools and their programs in the late-nineteenth century in a sense helped shape modern experimental biology negatively. In general, and like other academic sciences, biology was fundamentally reconstructed after the Civil War. In the process, it became infused with the American version of institutional concepts and scientific techniques coming from Europe. The field then gradually transitioned from a popularly and religiously oriented museum science of natural history to an academic discipline largely defined by laboratory research on animal form and function (Benson 1991). At Johns Hopkins University, for instance, "laboratory investigation, advanced instruction, and research in biology" "offered a new direction to the former natural history tradition" (ibid: 63). Philip Pauly argues that, apart from Johns Hopkins, where both medicine and biology were able to thrive next to each other, biology "prospered precisely" in regions where there was a "lack of sufficiently broad support for scientific medicine prior to 1900" (1984: 370). In other words, biology was able to maintain a strong position in those institutions (Harvard, Chicago, Columbia, or Pennsylvania, for example) in which the laboratory programs were not limited to or unable to provide for the practical preparation of medical students. Accordingly, protagonists in the biological field increasingly began to try and define the culture of experimental biology as the core of a general academic discipline that would organize and categorize the various specialties and subdisciplines that treated issues of organic nature. But their attempts to distinguish themselves culturally from their predecessors in the now outdated fields of natural history also had the effect of bringing the discipline of biology closer to that of medical science, where experimental practices had been propagated since the start of the nineteenth century in Europe and since the end of the Civil War in the USA.

Like the medical schools, biological departments in the last three decades of the nineteenth century also adopted the concept of the scientific method as a call "for a new approach to the teaching of science" (Benson 1991: 60). Just like their medical colleagues, they argued that students had to be exposed to nature directly through experiment, instead of being educated through the relay of natural phenomena in textbooks and lectures. They furthermore adopted the progressive understanding of the method described above. However, due to the lack of a professional recipient, such as sick patients for medicine, the ideology was reoriented toward the general goal of higher education and civic formation – something that hardly distinguished biology from general college education earlier in the century (Stichweh 1994a: 282f.). Biologists, like the medical scientific elite, therefore operated within the idea that the role of college training was to liberate the student from dogma and "discipline the mind" (Pauly 1984: 381). Biology would teach the methods and techniques of science "that students could use to deal 'scientifically' with problems of business, society, and politics" (ibid.). The shared cultural basis, however, led to attempts to distinguish the scientific sides of biology and medicine.

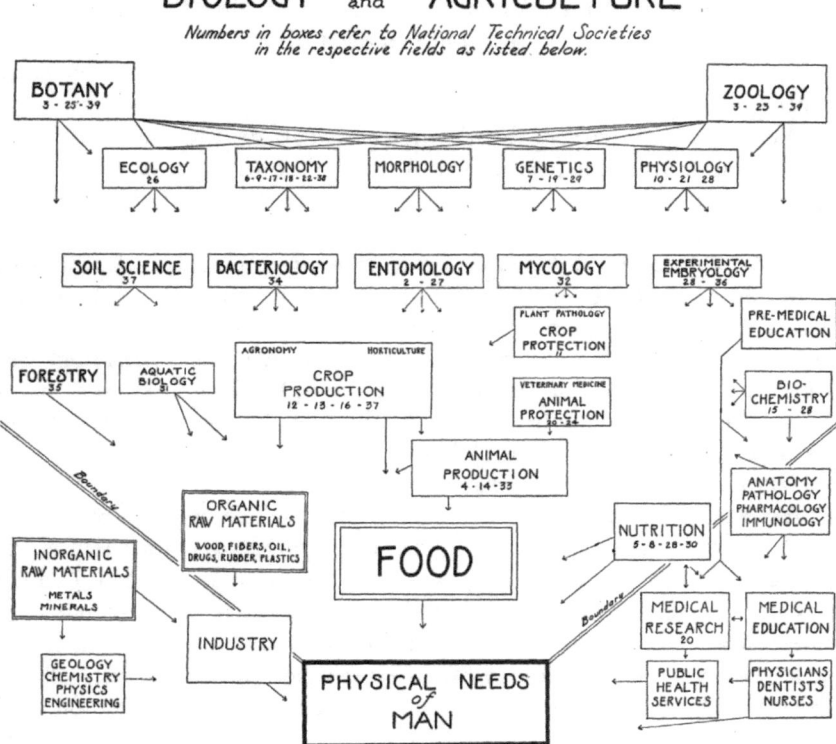

Figure 5.2: Organizational structure of biological and agricultural sciences in the USA in the 1940s, with botany and zoology as major cornerstones. Note that physiology is subsumed under zoology and other medical fields are separated by a boundary or situated at the fringes. I have omitted the list of societies that comes with the original image. (Source: Robert F. Griggs. 1942. The Organization of Biology and Agriculture. Science 96(2503). p. 546.)

Charles Whitman, for instance, founding director of the Marine Biological Laboratory in Woods Hole and professor in Chicago, promoted the idea of differentiating between morphology and physiology, and attacked the latter for being "limited too exclusively to the practical ends of medicine" (ibid: 384, see also Pauly 1987: 197). He was thus calling for the establishment of a "nonmedical 'biological physiology'", which was undistorted by medical concerns in concentrating on the organic functions of invertebrates (ibid.). Toward the end of the century, Jacques Loeb was beginning

157

to define an experimental area of "general physiology", which would later constitute a main element of academic biology in the US. He conceived of it as a comparative field of study, removed from any medical concerns, and with the explicit aim of solving "problems that would lead to scientific control over organisms" (Pauly 1987: 197).

The wording, however, already indicates that, despite the attempts to differentiate it from medicine, the institutional boundary between biological and medical work was becoming ambiguous. At some institutions the categorization "zoology" was preferred, instead of "biology", in order to verbally exclude the biological parts of medicine. But medical professors were nevertheless becoming "accustomed to university surroundings and began to encroach upon areas claimed by the biologists" (Pauly 1984: 388f.). At the same time, it was recognized that medicine's physiology was annexing turf in the "Pure Science and Philosophical faculties" and that it "should be placed and will be placed by the side of chemistry, physics, and the morphological division of biology" (ibid.).

Historian of science Toby Appel additionally shows that the founders of the American Physiological Society (APS), which was established in 1887, "were in effect appropriating the term 'physiology' for themselves" (Appel 1987: 166). Originally, physiology had a broad meaning, which was not restricted to the understanding of an experimental science as it emerged at the start of the nineteenth century in Europe. But the idea of an experimental physiology became representative of virtually all the "basic" medical sciences pursued in medical schools; and the physiological approaches to experimental investigations were also increasingly seen as relevant to morphological studies, which belonged, strictly speaking, to zoology (Fye 1987: 188f.). The science was framed as being experimental by the founding members of the association (all of them physicians by training, but with some of them having one foot also in natural history). Both the naturalists and the progressive medical community readily accepted this framing as the proper representation of physiology. "The new society by its membership policy, programs, and journal", Appel notes, "helped to define the discipline, at least in the early years, as experimental, medically-oriented animal physiology, neither too zoological nor too clinical" (1987: 166).

It requires no further explanation that the idea of a "medically-oriented" science left ample room for interpreting that orientation, so that the link to the actual institution of practical medicine was becoming weak. But as a scientific association, the interest of the APS was to make it as inclusive as possible for all who devoted themselves professionally to questions that fell within the purview of the ill-construed science of physiology. In short, people in both medical schools and natural sciences departments had to be included if they engaged in questions relevant for the APS and its community. Consequently, a shared research culture began to define work both in medical schools and biological departments.

After 1900, the situation became even more conflicting, as the culture of doing experimental work in biological and medical fields was no longer confined to the corresponding institutions but spread equally to medical schools and university departments. Zoologists assimilated the experimental techniques characteristic of physiological and biochemical research in the medical schools. But out of fear of incorporating "the alien culture of medical schools", they were reluctant to employ physiologists and biochemists (Kohler 1991: 313). Instead, at this point, medical schools were also harbouring scientists whose research interests were very remote from medicine, since "general physiologists found their best career chances in medical school departments of physiology and biochemistry" (ibid.).

Despite their colonization of medical school departments, biologists were nonetheless able to create a very narrowly defined disciplinary identity for their enterprise, with which they then began to settle on the fields of heredity and genetics to expand their constituencies into agriculture and industry (Pauly 1984: 394f.). But having been removed institutionally from the requirements of medical practice, the biological-medical culture of research began to establish itself in medical schools, without, however, the need of pursuing specifically medical interests. As I explain later in chapter 7, the molecular revolution in biology, for instance, took shape out of the biochemistry department at Stanford University's medical school. As a result, neither the territories nor the cultures of research devoted to these issues could be delineated neatly as biological or medical in the first decades of the twentieth century. Thus, while the new caste of clinical scientists began to distinguish themselves through their object of study, their academic territory, which was for them the phenomenon of disease as it appeared in the patient, scientists in the medical schools were left to devote themselves to more general questions about organic processes as they could be studied in animals – and later – other model organisms. However, at the same time, their relative freedom from clinical concerns and the early formative stage of modern academic biology in the US led to ambiguities between medical science and the communities of experimental biological researchers. On the level of research policy, this was paving the way for later conflicts over the funding of research fields (Appel 2000).

6. Constructing the Identity of a Late Modern Discipline – Biomedical Science and the Life Sciences in the Post-War United States

In science and technology studies (STS) and adjacent fields, the concept of biomedicine is presented as a new medical paradigm based on the molecular understanding of bodily functions. However, it is also enlisted as an example to argue against the prevailing science policy ideology of the postwar era – the so-called linear model of innovation and the concepts of basic and applied research. In this context, biomedicine epitomizes a distinctly technoscientific understanding that refers to complex transformations of the epistemological, material and institutional configurations of medicine and science in the late-twentieth century (Clarke et al. 2003, see also Keating/Cambrosio 2003). Basic and applied research became prominent during the restructuring of US science policy after World War II and have since determined much of the logic of modern research (Schauz 2014). The corresponding linear model of innovation constitutes a conceptual framework to comprehend the relation of science and technology to the economy, stating that innovation starts with basic research, moving through applied research to development and dissemination (Godin 2006).

The postwar notions of the linear model and of basic/applied research have come under sharp attack in the STS community more generally starting in the 1990s. Authors here have denied the empirical and analytical significance of basic research, relating it to nineteenth-century pure science ideals and placing it against the backdrop of claims that the scientific system has undergone profound changes since the end of the twentieth century (e.g., Gibbons et al. 1992). These changes are taken to signal a paradigm shift, as Schauz recounts, in which "application-oriented research programmes with cooperative and transdisciplinary project teams have replaced the former university-centered basic research" (2014: 274). In this regard, social and cultural studies of biomedicine highlight the category as signifying a new system of interdisciplinary practices, in which the biological and medical laboratory as well as the clinic have moved together due to the molecularization and automation of processes. Peter Keating and Alberto Cambrosio (2003), for instance, use biomedicine as an analytical category that describes scientific practices particularly prevalent in research hospitals of the second half of the twentieth century. They and other authors deny that the category of biomedicine – in the sense of the linear model and basic and applied research – equals the "one-way application of laboratory studies to therapeutics" (Scheffler/Strasser 2015: 664).

I contend, though, that upon closer inspection, this thesis is supported mainly by the employment of sort of a historiographical straw man. I want to explain this with the undifferentiated use of the term "scientific medicine" (which I discussed at the start of chapter 4) to signify virtually all forms of academic medicine preceding the era of biomedicine. This argument abstracts from much of the sematic heritage, which – as I will show here – comes *neither* from postwar clinical medicine and hospital discourses, nor from discussions of the technoscientification of medicine at the end of the twentieth century. Instead, the idea of biomedicine emerged from the research policy debates on basic and applied research after World War II, i.e., from precisely the context from which biomedicine is in the literature taken to be a departure. The assertion is that, in contrast to previous decades, molecular technologies have significantly improved the relationship between the laboratory and the clinic. Therefore, against the linear understanding, "practical" investigations in the hospital are said to contribute no less to the production of "knowledge about the workings of disease and their possible treatment than experiments in laboratories" (Scheffler/Strasser 2015: 664, see also Keating/Cambrosio 2004).[67]

I have illustrated, though, that such supposedly only biomedical conditions were present already in the concept of scientific medicine in Germany and that also the clinical science of the early-twentieth century USA can be regarded as a category that distanced itself from the mechanical ideals of physiological therapeutics, i.e., the almost automatic one-way application of laboratory science to the treatment of disease. Accordingly, in this chapter, I want to show that biomedicine does not necessarily denote a new medical paradigm of the late-twentieth century, but that instead it was devised as a new way of categorizing work in medical and biological research in the postwar era. The concept was prominently employed in the US science policy discourse at a moment in time when it became necessary to reorganize research in biology and medicine due to the changing institutional structures and the vast expansion of the science funding system

---

67 In a now classic study, Löwy (1996), for instance, shows how it was crucial that also clinicians and patients contributed to the making of interleukin II as a cancer agent in France. She details the processes of research and intervention that took place between the ward and the clinical laboratory.

after the war. The idea of biomedicine was introduced into this context through the shorthand "biomedical", and the label "biomedical science" grouped work on basic biological mechanisms conducted both in university departments and medical schools to distinguish it from other fields in the so-called "life sciences" (US Senate 1959), which had no immediate relevance for public health.

However, as I argue, the distinction was not due to epistemic or practical differences between biomedical science and the rest of the life sciences. Rather, reasons were much more mundane and concerned the administration of research activities in the United States. Nevertheless, through the restructuring of medical and biological sciences in the postwar era the category came to transport specific promises about the relationship between bench research and bedside practice, which I call the "linear legacy" of biomedicine. What is striking is that, in this context, the linear understanding of biomedicine, which sociologists and historians dealing with the topic reject, was engrained into the category as a central feature. Actors in the post-war United States rendered biomedicine – *qua* biomedical science – an autonomous scientific discipline that laid the theoretical basis for future health care improvements. These promises, in turn, need to be understood as deriving from the implications made by actors during the processes of disciplinary reconstruction. The category was used to define a broad scientific culture, which had established itself in academic institutions that were originally distinct, as I demonstrated earlier, namely, in university natural science departments and medical schools.

Consequently, the dimension of my analysis shifts somewhat with the investigation of biomedicine. While previous chapters explored ideas of local research cultures, or the relationship between academic tribes and territories, biomedicine constitutes sort of a meta-discipline like modern day chemistry or biology, comprising many heterogenous research cultures. What now becomes dominant for making a disciplinary identity is what I described as "global narratives of science" in chapter 2, i.e., the visions and expectations of how a science will contribute to improvements in society. I will therefore demonstrate how biomedicine's underlying linear legacy can be attributed to the ideological power exerted by the concept of basic research in the postwar era. The idea of basic research emerged as part of a larger science policy scheme, in which the notion of a linear relationship between scientific research and its application was dominant. In the context of biomedicine, this led to the idea that the crucial dynamic between research and medical practice was that *from* laboratory bench *to* clinical bedside (Kraft 2013: 29). The linear expectations for innovations associated with biomedicine allowed the community of basic researchers to (re-)establish or maintain a connection to the community of clinical medicine. This connection had largely been dissolved conceptually through the reorganization of medical science in the early decades of the twentieth century and during the war.

To understand the meaning of biomedicine, therefore, it requires taking seriously how the category was employed in the post-war discourse. In this context, as I will show, the term emerged as part of a larger scheme in the reconstruction of US research policy, in which the ideology of a linear relationship between scientific research and its application was indeed prevalent. The focus of actors active in defining key concepts in the period under consideration accordingly changed from institution building to the maintenance of the already established structures. Traditional disciplinary and institutional boundaries in the biological and medical sciences, as we saw, were losing their relevance for science policy at the start of the century, due to a shift to research project-oriented distinctions. However, the war effort had contributed considerably to the general growth of science. To counter the ambiguity of biological and medical activities that was looming since the start of the century, actors saw the need to design a coherent national research policy that would cover both basic laboratory research with and without prospects for medical case.

I want to show how policy makers in the post-war era engaged in a form of boundary work (Gieryn 1999) to legitimize the existence of the broad research culture, which had developed in parallel in medical schools and biology departments. The boundary work approach describes demarcation processes based on the discursive attribution and usurpation of epistemic authority with respect to actors and practices. In my context, to distinguish biomedical from other biological activities, the boundary that was drawn concerned the attribution and usurpation of these research activities with reference to a health care mission. I argue that the young but already existing category of the life sciences – initially synonymous with biomedical science – proved unsuitable as a scientific category. The life sciences comprised a row of biological research activities, experimental and natural-historic, as well as research conducted under roof of medical schools. The reason for the category's unsuitableness, however, was not because it defined the disciplinary culture of those activities inadequately, but because it put them under the purview of the National Science Foundation (NSF) (US Senate 1959). The NSF grew out of the reigning new ideology of basic science as the patron for disinterested and curiosity-driven research

(Kaldewey/Schauz 2018: 124f.). Funding research in medical schools with an interest of health care would have openly betrayed that commitment.

The National Institutes of Health (NIH), however, emerged as the by far largest supporter of basic biological research after the war. As the name states, the institute has an obvious health care-oriented mission. However, it would have been highly inconsistent in keeping with the prevailing basic/applied science distinction to classify all the research under the NIH's patronage as applied vis-à-vis the basic research under the NSF's custody. Consequently, in a 1965 official report on the activities of the NIH, the term "biomedical science" crystalized (NIH Study Committee 1965). It was previously employed as a shorthand for grouping research in biology and medicine in other government agencies and allowed to superimpose the basic/applied distinction with the orientation towards agency mission. The new category thus met both the linguistic requirements of science policy and of the situation of federal research funding after the war. It also defined the scientific cultures that had developed in parallel in various institutions of biology and medicine as a discipline of research activities with a broader health care-mission, in contradistinction to that conducted without the explicit medical relevance.

I. The Birth of the Administrative Shorthand "Biomedical"

To understand how the meaning of biomedicine was made and endowed with a linear legacy, I want to first clear up some issues about when and how the category was introduced and subsequently used in the postwar discourse. Many scholars point to its initial mentioning in the 1923 edition of *Dorland's Illustrated Medical Dictionary*, where it is defined as "clinical medicine based on the principles of physiology and biochemistry". While this seems to be a rather conservative rendering, which could have originated with physiological therapeutics or similar movements, there is need for caution with the use of sources here, especially since most of the scholars in question seem to draw on Keating's and Cambrosio's well-informed etymological elaborations of the term (2003: 51ff., see also Bruchhausen 2011: 499f., Quirke/Gaudillière 2008: 445, Scheffler/Strasser 2015: 663, Strasser 2014: 11). However, Keating and Cambrosio themselves alertly present the entry as tied up in a "case of self-reference", in which "the source of the *Dorland's* definition remains unknown" (ibid: 52). They nonetheless argue for the significance of the early coinage of the term, although "we can find only isolated instances of the word prior to World War II" (ibid.).

But it seems easy to overestimate the importance of the purported early appearance, since the category only entered into general usage around mid-century. Since the start of the twentieth century, and considerably accelerated by the war effort, traditional disciplinary and institutional boundaries in the biological and medical sciences were losing relevance for making science policy. The introduction of the concept of basic science, which became prominent after the war ended, only accelerated the disregard for such differentiations. This situation is reflected in the fact that neither government agencies like the NIH, which was founded on the clear mission of sponsoring research with health-related content, nor the NSF, which understood itself as a patron of basic research, differentiated between whether funds were going to medical schools or to university departments of the natural sciences, nor between disciplines traditionally associated with either biology or medicine.[68] As a consequence, based on questions of what distinguished health-related and non-health-related basic research projects, policy makers and their scientific advisors in the period from the end of the war to the 1960s engaged in attempts to clearly define the different research activities in biology and medicine for the sake of formulating a coherent science policy (Appel 2000, see also Keating/Cambrosio 2003: 56, Schauz 2014: 302f.).[69]

After the war, the notion of biomedicine began to constitute a neat umbrella term for much of basic research in biology and medicine that would yield potential future applications in the clinic. However, it was the adjective "biomedical", not the noun "biomedicine", which was first referred to as a categorization of scientific work in the US research policy discourse of the postwar period (figure 6.2). Not only was the noun not yet widely used at the time, but the fashion in which federal agencies employed the adjective is in accordance with the way in which the term became popularized through the concept of "biomedical science" in later tensions between the NIH and the NSF.

---

68 They inherited this approach of funding especially from the Rockefeller Foundation's initiative to fund short-term project-oriented instead of disciplinary affiliated research (Schneider 2015).

69 As such, the category biomedicine is part of a more general transition in science and politics denoted by the appearance of new vocabulary to legitimate new forms of doing and organizing research after World War II (Kaldewey 2013: 364, Schauz 2014: 299).

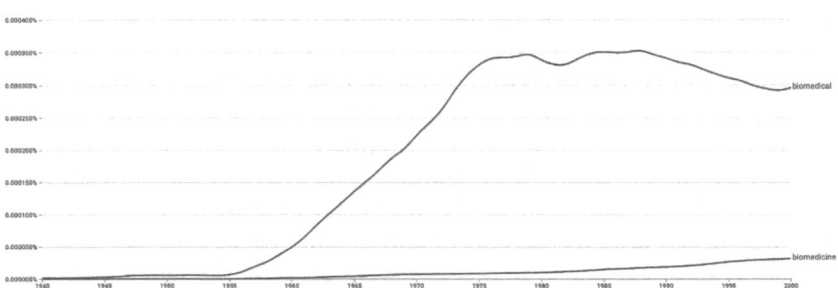

Figure 6.1: Word frequency of "biomedical" and "biomedicine", 1940–2000. (Source: Google Books Ngram Viewer, https://books.google.com/ngrams/graph?co ntent=biomedicine%2Cbiomedical&year_start=1940&year_end=2000&cor pus=26&smoothing=3. [Accessed November 22, 2021]).

Rather than taking the noun to constitute a new form of scientific and medical practice,[70] the term needs to be understood as originating from a shorthand for describing agency divisions, which were active both in biological and medical research in the early decades after the war. In 1948, for instance, the term was used to describe a health division at the Atomic Energy Commission (AEC), which ran studies on the pathological reactions of living organisms to extreme environments like nuclear fallout. "Although the group was alternatively known as the 'Biological and Medical Research Group,'" Keating and Cambrosio aptly note, "the first annual report (1949) of the Health Division used the term 'Biomedical Research Group' and would routinely do so in subsequent reports" (Keating/Cambrosio 2003: 354, n. 31). The National Aeronautics and Space Administration (NASA) ran similar "biomedical" studies in the late-1950s, but with a focus on how living organisms reacted in outer space, before "the 1960s ushered in the first official reports on biomedicine [sic] and the organization of international meetings" devoted to the subject (Keating/Cambrosio 2003: 56). Subsequently, the term appeared in writings

---

70 Keating and Cambrosio also acknowledge the peculiarities of the category in an endnote to their book, explaining how usually the noun of a word enters circulation before an adjective is derived from it and becomes used. But "[b]ecause of the prior existence of both 'medicine' and 'biology,' this is probably not the case for 'biomedicine'." They also point out that "in some languages the term 'biomedical' has had a career independent of the substantive 'biomedicine'" (2003: 352, n. 9).

about the medical aspects in engineering, computer science as well as statistics and mathematics (Bruchhausen 2010: 499).

In other words, against the backdrop of the convergence of research work in biological and medical departments since the early twentieth century, AEC and NASA administrators around mid-century thought it convenient to express this convergence in the official documents they drafted – most likely unaware of the far-reaching consequences this would have for the later organization of the natural and medical sciences. Thus, even if *Dorland's* constituted a solid source, we could disregard its definition of biomedicine: the noun developed only after its meaning had already been defined by the shorthand adjective. Furthermore, if the noun was not yet widely used in the 1940s and 1950s, we can only speculate whether agency administrators took notice of it when devising their version. Therefore, their use of the term in government administration must be seen as constituting the semantic origin of biomedicine, rather than the clinical medicine meaning of *Dorland's*.

II. *From "Allied" to "Underlying" Sciences*

Having sorted out the etymology of the prevalent basic concept, I can now turn to the specifics of how actors came to employ the category, following a period of far-reaching reconceptualization in science policy. It is known that the idea of basic science effectively replaced the older ideal of pure science as the dominant category after the end of World War II, although this did not mean that it simply adopted the meaning of the former category (Kaldewey 2013: 360–371, Schauz 2014: 298–313). In his famous report to US President Harry S. Truman in 1945, titled "Science – The Endless Frontier", Vannevar Bush (1995) used the concept to legitimize new forms of doing and organizing research, particularly the continuation in peacetime of the large-scale public support for scientific research begun during the war. While the pure science ideal meant that the pursuit of science was imbued with moral qualities, Bush's "basic research", in contrast, received its importance through helping to achieve the larger goal of social progress (Kaldewey/Schauz 2018: 110–116, 122–129). The report justified government expenditure for basic research on the grounds of arguing that advancing medical research would enhance public health; that more research would lead to prosperity, due to economic growth, job security and the availability of new technologies; and that it would guarantee a technological advantage of the USA's armaments over its enemies (particularly the Soviet Union). "Only then", according to Désirée Schauz, "did basic research become a real keyword in research funding. And the metaphor of 'basic' did the trick; by laying the basics for all kinds of future benefits, the federal government financed basic research as for the common good" (2014: 299).

However, the new category solidified by Bush's report conflicted with the cultural and institutional distinctions that existed in biology and medicine, and therefore, in the long run, warranted a new category to classify basic research activities directed toward the larger goal of public health. The conceptual conflicts become apparent through comparison of the vocabulary of Bush's report with the older terminology used to characterize medical science since the turn from the nineteenth to the twentieth century. The dominant framing until about the end of the war was "medicine and allied sciences".[71] This use of terminology can be explained with the institutional rearrangements that characterised scientific medicine in the early decades of the twentieth century. Allied sciences were those natural sciences supporting the furthering of medical knowledge, like biochemistry or microbiology. Since medical science as an institution had become removed from clinical medicine through the establishment of its own clinical science discipline, the scientific basis of medicine began to be defined more by its allegiance to the other experimental sciences rather than to medical practice. It therefore seems to be no coincidence that Samuel Meltzer, for example, one of the chief inventors of the pure science of clinical medicine, already employed the phrase at an early point. That the concept was also still popular in the science policy discourses immediately after the war can be drawn from a document published in 1947, "Science and Public Policy" (the so-called Steelman-Report), designed to assess for the US President the situation in science and research.

Volume five of the report, "The Nation's Medical Research", refers to the concept throughout in different variations (Steelman 1947: iii, 3, 4, 6, 10, 13, 15, 17, 18, 19, 20, 24, 27, 30, 73, 93, 96, 101, 108, 113, 114).[72] The concept clearly implied an equal footing of medicine and other biological laboratory disciplines in the context of the pure science ideal, but

---

71 The Department of the History of Medicine at Yale University, for example, still referenced the old terminology, when launching the *Journal of the History of Medicine and Allied Sciences*, which published its first issue in January 1946, https://academic.oup.com/jhmas (accessed November 22, 2021).

72 Next to "medicine and allied sciences", the report uses mainly the words "medical and allied research", "research in medical and allied fields", or "medical and allied sciences", thereby underscoring their commonalities as sciences.

it referred to them as housed under the roof of the medical school – it included fields like physiology, pathology, bacteriology, biochemistry or pharmacology. Accordingly, the "allied sciences" meant only a limited number of "biological" fields in total. And I illustrated in the previous chapter that physiology was a broad and ambiguous field appropriated also by biologists.

Before the 1940s, biology was still divided into three major and institutionally largely separate groups. Botany and zoology formed the major disciplines that were, for the most part, organized in separate departments at American universities (see also figure 5.3). The other group of important "'biological' disciplines – anatomy, physiology, biochemistry" – had their home almost exclusively in the medical schools. "They had their own departments, doctoral programs, societies, and journals; they scarcely interacted with botany and zoology" (Appel 2000: 14). For the time being, the institutional separation held. The notion of "medicine and the allied sciences" was still able to circumscribe fields housed in the medical school as opposed to university departments of biology (i.e., botany and zoology). However, as I indicated earlier, with the reform of medical schools, turning them into genuinely academic institutions at the start of the twentieth century, ambiguities were looming with respect to the description of medical and biological research.

Additionally, the general format of research funding changed after the Great Crash of 1923, since private philanthropies were hit hard by the following economic depression. Until World War II, private philanthropies shouldered the major burden of promoting research. The Rockefeller Foundation, founded in 1913, was the largest private philanthropy to sponsor medicine and science in the early decades of the twentieth century. Initially, the program of the foundation was directed towards broad areas like education and public health. But the economic situation compelled a reorganization of the institution. The reorganization meant, among other things, that the "broad goal of 'welfare of mankind'" changed into the "narrower focus of 'the advancement of knowledge'" (Schneider 2015: 286, see also Kohler 1991: 239ff.). Accordingly, the foundation's Division of Medical Education turned into that of Medical Science and was situated next to the divisions for the natural sciences, the social science and the humanities. The Rockefeller Foundation's subsequent emphasis was now on supporting research (admittedly, the creation of academic medical institutions had from the start also implied giving money for laboratory investigations). In the process, the institution adopted a new practice of patronage and turned "from institution building to aiding individual projects in specific research fields", as Kohler notes (1991: 260, see also Schneider 2015: 287).

More importantly, however, this added to the ambiguity between biological and medical research because grants for biological projects were also going to researchers in medical schools (Kohler 1991: 313–321). The new concept of the project grant conflicted with common practices of distinguishing between biology and medicine institutionally. Research projects were now being supported based on their specific problem formulation and not on the grounds of their institutional location. The introduction of the project grant mechanism into science policy signals the emerging importance of research as a central quality of disciplinary cultures (Kaldewey/Schauz 2018: 116f.). For medicine, this meant a shift from methods and practices to making original discoveries. Scientists, in both university departments of the natural sciences and in medical schools, were beginning to pursue research work in "general physiology", which could be associated with medicine as well as with animal morphology. They began to communicate professionally with each other over problems of their research and began forming a community that was undertaking their work neither strictly for clinical nor zoological interests.

The institutional separation of medical and biological research practices was further undermined by the rhetoric in Bush's own account to the President and the post-war situation of federal research expenditure. As Appel (2000) shows in her insightful book about the NSF and the constitution of biology in the post-war United States, the US government contributed only a limited amount to the support of biological research or to medical research and education before World War II. During the war, the US Office of Scientific Research and Development's (OSRD) Committee on Medical Research became the chief resource for funding projects in medical science, while the patronage of private foundations receded dramatically in comparison. "The federal government provided lavish support not only for physicians' clinical investigations but also for research in such medically related fields as physiology, biochemistry, and pharmacology" (ibid: 14). Purely biological studies, in contrast, were left virtually unsupported by the Office at the time. After the war, however, the NIH, which was formally established in 1930, had taken over a stock of project contracts from the OSRD. These contracts did not adhere to the institutional distinction between medical schools and university departments, thereby effectively establishing the NIH as a key player in patronage of research in both medical and biological disciplines (Appel 2000: 32, see also Swain 1962: 1235).

This change is also reflected in the introduction of a uniform ideology of basic science equally to all fields. Therefore, where there used to be institutional distinctions regarding disciplinary cultures, Bush no longer differentiated between the university and the medical school:

"The primary place for medical research is in the medical schools *and* universities. [...] Apart from teaching, however, the primary obligation of the medical schools *and* universities is to continue the traditional function of such institutions, namely, to provide the individual worker with an opportunity for free, untrammeled study of nature, in the directions and by the methods suggested by his interests, curiosity, and imagination. The history of medical science teaches clearly the supreme importance of affording the prepared mind complete freedom for the exercise of initiative. It is the special province of the medical schools *and* universities to foster medical research in this way – a duty which cannot be shifted to Government agencies, industrial organizations, or to any other institutions" (1995: 15, my emphasis).

With institutional differences becoming irrelevant for categorizing research, the relationship between medicine and its allied sciences shifted significantly. While they were once convened within the walls of the medical schools, they were now categorically joined with other biological fields across institutional divides. The direct responsibility for clinical medicine had become the task of the clinical science discipline. Consequently, the basic biological and medical sciences, in concordance with the basic science ideology, became subordinate to the larger goal of public health. Their task was not with clinical practice but has been ever since with laying the knowledge foundations for future improvements in health care. Hence, Bush no longer spoke of medicine and its "allied sciences" in his report,[73] as if they were equal fields in the same institution. Instead, in keeping with the "basic" metaphor also here, he substituted the concept for the term "underlying sciences":

"It is wholly probable that progress in the treatment of cardiovascular disease, renal disease, cancer, and similar refractory diseases will be made as the result of fundamental discoveries in subjects unrelated to those diseases, and perhaps entirely unexpected by the investigator.

---

73 The phrase "medicine and allied sciences" appears only in the letter of transmittal of the Chairman of the Medical Advisory Board to Bush, included in the 1960-edition of "Science – The Endless Frontier" (Bush 1995: 47).

[...] Progress in the war against disease results from discoveries in remote and unexpected fields of medicine and the *underlying sciences*. Further progress requires that the entire front of medicine and the *underlying sciences* of chemistry, physics, anatomy, biochemistry, physiology, pharmacology, bacteriology, pathology, parasitology, etc., be broadly developed" (ibid: 14, my emphasis).

Bush's conceptualization of the relationship between medicine and science greatly expanded the spectrum of sciences that would be seen as able to contribute to the improvement of public health well beyond the confines of the original scientific discipline of medicine. But it also defined them as remote to, or even detached from, the actual concerns of clinical practice. This contributed to the removal of an inherited responsibility for practical medicine, which seemed to rest now more with clinical science, and it also lowered the stakes for those who wished to frame their work as a contribution to the nation's health. I will discuss later that this ambiguity about the responsibilities for clinical matters becomes especially pressing, when biomedicine is used not as the name for a basic science discipline, but as an overarching supercategory to designate all of the academic health care system, including clinical science and practice.[74]

At the same time, while the new terminology left the integrity of such mentioned disciplines as physics or chemistry intact, it had a noticeable effect on the social identity of biology, which was aiming to establish itself as a unified and autonomous field after World War II. If neither institutional nor disciplinary boundaries could any longer guarantee a differentiation between research pursued for the end of improving public health and research conducted for the sake of expanding the knowledge of biological forms and functions, it required the invention of new research policy categories, which could draw a clear boundary to prevent that biology's disciplinary identity would be appropriated by a dependence on medical ends.

---

74 Today, the term biomedicine is largely used as a supercategory to describe the academic health care system globally. It defines the bridging of laboratory research and clinical practice. But in the science policy discourses after World War II, biomedical science was understood as a basic research discipline that only laid the foundations for the possibilities of future improvements in public health. In the conclusion to my book, I will reflect on some of the implications this ambiguity in meaning has for our society's understanding of science and medicine.

III. The Political Boundary Between Biomedical Science and the Life Sciences

There existed a term – "life sciences" – with the potential to define the different cultures of basic experimental research as a disciplinary community, as a report commissioned by the US Senate and published in 1959, titled "The National Science Foundation and the Life Sciences", reveals (US Senate 1959). The plural form of the word "science", however, indicates that it was still only a loose bracket around a larger multidisciplinary field, which included work being done in medical school laboratories (figure 6.2). The NSF established a joint Division of Biological and Medical Sciences in 1952. Appel reports that Alan Waterman, the NSF's first appointed director, proclaimed that the agency did not make any distinction "programwise between basic research in the medical sciences and basic research in the biological sciences" (Appel 2000: 52, see also US Senate 1959: 1, 15). Instead, research in these areas was supported based on distinguishing biological functions.

Field	1st year	Intermediate	Terminal year	Total by field
Life sciences:				
Agriculture	1	2	2	5
Anthropology	2	7	5	14
Biochemistry	8	20	8	36
Biophysics	4	6	1	11
Botany	8	5	7	20
General biology	2	4	1	7
Genetics	1	12	4	17
Medical sciences	4	9	2	15
Microbiology	5	2	4	11
Psychology	8	18	4	30
Zoology	22	37	25	84
Total, life sciences	65	122	63	250

Figure 6.2: *Example of the grouping of research fields under the rubric 'life sciences' in the Senate report on the NSF. Botany, zoology as well as medical sciences feature as part of the category. The table refers to the distribution of predoctoral awards of the NSF offered by scientific field and year, 1958–59. (Source: United States Senate. 1959. The National Science Foundation and the Life Sciences. Washington, D.C.: The US Government. p. 35; https://books.google. de/books?id=rZVUAAAAMAAJ&printsec=frontcover&hl=de&source=gbs_ge _summary_r&cad=0#v=onepage&q&f=false [accessed November 22, 2021]).*

The Foundation accordingly had programs for the support of basic research organized around eight categories: "(1) developmental biology; (2) environmental biology; (3) genetic biology; (4) metabolic biology; (5) molecular biology; (6) psychobiology; (7) regulatory biology; and (8) systematic biology" (US Senate 1959: 2, 13ff., see also Appel 2000: 64ff.). Conceiving of basic research in this fashion was the result of new ways of approaching biological problems that had developed since the 1930s. Warren Weaver of the Rockefeller Foundation, for example, introduced the idea of grouping biological research according to the overarching idea of "vital processes" instead of disciplinary demarcations, whereby he fostered a field of biological science that also harboured physicists and chemists (Kohler 1991: 275–283).

While a focus on biological function helped establish new areas of research, by the 1940s it also caused the traditional barriers, which separated botanists and zoologists, and biological researchers in university departments and in medical schools, to crumble (Appel 2000: 16). As Appel attentively notes, the distinction into the functional categories allowed for the NSF to support their own version of basic research in medicine, "since biomedical [sic] categories were effectively hidden under biological rubrics" (ibid: 64). As decreed by its founding document, the NSF understood itself as a federal patron for sciences that contributed to the general expansion of knowledge – the "endless frontier" – as a foundation for social progress. Regarding medicine and biology, the term "life" aptly reflects this broad comprehension. Supported programs encompassed the areas of biological, medical and agricultural sciences and "conceived basic research in the life sciences so that biological processes, whether in plant, animal, or man," were "seen in their basic contexts" (US Senate 1959: 13).

However, the two major federal agencies – the NIH and the NSF – were competing over funding these activities at the start of the post-war era. It appeared incongruous that the NSF, as the patron of the prestigious category of basic science, was factually being dwarfed by the NIH, which despite its clear mission, was providing funding to basic research in biological fields. Therefore, drawing a clear distinction between jurisdictions of both agencies became a matter of utmost political importance. Actors used the method of emphasizing the differences in mission that was attached to the NSF and the NIH for this purpose.[75] The criterion that was being used to distinguish the NSF's program in the life sciences from other federal agencies was that it was not "subject to the limitations, however broad, of a specific program commitment or assigned mission" (ibid: viii). The NSF was seeking a hegemony over basic research-patronage, while at the

---

75 Next to the NIH, other agencies that competed for financing research in the life sciences in the period, which included the Office of Naval research and the AEC (Appel 2000: 24–30).

same time trying to avoid duplication with other funding agencies (Appel 2000: 101–129). The only viable strategy regarding the NIH – which was the most serious competitor in the business of federally funding research in the life sciences – was for NSF protagonists to try and draw a clear line between the sort of activities conducted under the support of the NSF and the NIH.

Accordingly, Waterman explained in the preface to the 1960-edition of "Science – The Endless Frontier" what distinguished the two agencies:

> "The National Institutes of Health stresses research aimed at the care and cure of diseases, including basic research related to its mission, as defined by Executive Order 10512. The National Science Foundation, on the other hand, supports basic research in this area primarily for the purpose of advancing our knowledge and understanding of biological and medical fields" (Waterman 1995: xii).

But how precisely was basic research "related to the cure and care of disease" different from basic research "for the purpose of advancing our knowledge and understanding of biological and medical fields"? In both cases, the concept of basic research defines "research performed without thought of practical ends" (Bush 1995: 18)? To put it crudely, if concrete practical outcomes for the clinic were not the measure by which to distinguish the missions of both agencies, adherence to either of them appeared to amount to not much more than paying lip service. It depended on the communicative framing of how research work would potentially pay-off in either one or the other direction – a communication that could be adapted strategically and in accordance with where funds were coming from. I will explain in the next chapter how molecular biologists jumped the biomedical bandwagon by employing the appropriate communicative framing to their research projects.

Like the sciences supported by the NSF, the NIH's purview in the post-war period also encompassed a broad range of activities that could not inherently be reduced to their health care implications. But to make its health-related mission more visible, the organization was restructured after the war from being based on medical disciplines to overseeing disease categories (Park 2008). Actors campaigning in support of the NSF took advantage of the NIH's new categorization in attempts to frame the agency as better suited to support research conducted on the "applied" side of science rather than in genuinely basic areas. Their hope was that this framing would reflect on how the federal government allocated its budget to the agencies. Maintaining that applied research was already receiving its full share, it was therefore not more applied, but basic research that was needed to ensure medical progress. This argument implied nothing else than that the government should stock up the budget of the NSF for basic research in the according fields and not that of the NIH (Appel 2000: 106, see also 116f.).

According to the Senate-commissioned report on the NSF and the life sciences, unbound scientific curiosity and creativity was viewed as the main quality sought for through basic research in biological and medical sciences, as opposed to "immediate and practical results" (US Senate 1959: ix, see also Bush 1995: 12). "The subcommittee [of the Senate] has welcomed the many affirmations of this sound concept of encouraging creativity on the part of the Federal organization most directly concerned with research against disease – the National Institutes of Health" (ibid.). Therefore, while not directly denying the NIH its legitimacy of receiving a budget for supporting basic research, the disease category-structure of the NIH was nevertheless used to indirectly create a hierarchy between the two agencies, to assign them separate jurisdictions in the realm of biological and medical sciences:

> "But, sometimes, rigidity of procedure creates a paradox: (*a*) we increase resources for applied, i.e. *categorical*, medical research (and very justifiably so, in my personal judgment). But, simultaneously, (*b*) we deny desperately needed and urgently requested resources to expand *pure* [sic] research proportionately.
> The result is that pure research is still a stepchild, receiving what constitutes but a small fraction of the total. The culprit responsible for this paradox is the 'either-or' way of thinking. Surely, we should have learned by now that *both* pure and applied research are essential." (ibid: x)

However, despite arguments that disease categories downgraded the NIH to an agency that was better suited to foster applied research, they were a factor that did not only play into the hands of those seeking to establish the NSF as the main patron for basic research in all biological and medical fields. Historian Buhm Soon Park has looked closely at the development of the NIH's intramural and extramural funding programs in the post-war period. He notes that disease categories constituted a concept ambiguous enough to rhetorically serve the promotion of a variety of research activities – basic and applied, medical and biological – under the heading of benefitting the future health care of society. He argues in fact "that there was a common goal among the categorical institutes at the NIH to establish a strong *basic research* program covering several scientific fields, even if their links to categorical missions might be neither direct nor transparent" (Park 2008: 28, my emphasis). At any rate, next to research grants awarded according to the categorical division of the NIH's institutes, the agency also reserved money for support of non-categorical research. This practice was manifested by the creation of, first, in 1958, a Division, and later, in 1962, an Institute of General Medical Sciences. Accordingly, the mandate of the NIH expanded beyond research oriented towards specific diseases and also encompassed activities that fell inside the NSF's jurisdiction over the life sciences. As a result, by the 1960s, the NIH was funding research in virtually all life science areas and responsible for the largest share in federal support of professional biologists (Appel 2000: 138ff.).

Subsuming the work not only of biologically oriented medical researchers but also of biologists under federal health research policy meant that the term "life sciences" was unable to adequately capture the differences that constituted the activities of the NSF and the NIH. It therefore required an additional category, a similar umbrella term coming from the side of medicine. This term needed to draw the boundary between forms of research under purview of agencies with a mandate to support science for the broader societal outlook and those that had a more narrowly defined health-related goal – albeit these pursuits were hardly distinguishable when looking at their research cultures. A study committee, chaired by Dean Wooldridge and appointed by the White House to examine the activities of the NIH was to deliver the necessary semantic specification. Published in 1965, the report to President Lyndon B. Johnson by the Woolridge-Committee was titled "Biomedical Science and Its Administration", employing the administrative shorthand, which agencies like the AEC and NASA had previously used for categorizing their inhouse research (NIH Study Committee 1965, see also figure 6.3). The report is generally credited with having relayed the category to a larger audience and with defining the modern enterprise publicly (Bruchhausen 2010: 499f., see also Keating/Cambrosio 2004: 364f.).

To be sure, the report does not set out to explicitly define "biomedical science". Instead, the language of the report reveals how the adjective "biomedical" was already an accepted vocabulary in US science policy discourses by the time it was written, because of the AEC and NASA. Originally, it implied something very similar to the term life sciences, namely, the convenient grouping of basic research in biological and medical fields under one heading. The above-mentioned report by the Senate Subcommittee (published six years prior to the Woolridge-Report), for instance, had also employed the adjective. In the Letter of Transmittal by the chairman – and only here – the term biomedical research is used. It acts as a synonym for basic research in the life sciences, in order to state the purpose of the report as to summarize the activities of the NSF that bear on the fields of biology and medicine (US Senate 1959: iii).

BIOMEDICAL SCIENCE

AND ITS

ADMINISTRATION,

A Study of The National Institutes of Health

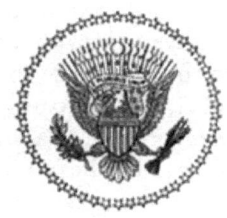

THE WHITE HOUSE

WASHINGTON, D.C.

FEBRUARY 1965

Figure 6.3: Title page to the Wooldridge Report "Biomedical Science and its Administration. A Study of the National Institutes of Health", The White House, Washington D.C., released February 1965, which made "biomedical science" an official concept in science policy discourses (Source: Google Books, https://boo ks.google.de/books?id=cK0wAAAAIAAJ&printsec=frontcover&hl=de&source =gbs_ge_summary_r&cad=0#v=onepage&q&f=false [accessed November 22, 2021).

The Woolridge-Report describes the NIH's conception of science as implying the same basic science-ideology that was at the heart of the NSF:

> "In general terms, the public funds that support NIH activities are intended to 'buy' for the American people a commensurate degree of relief from suffering and improvement of health. To achieve this goal, NIH devotes its principal effort to a broad program of investigation of life processes, rather than to a search for direct cure or prevention of specific diseases. It employs this approach for a simple and valid reason: life science is so complex, and what is known about fundamental biological processes is so little, that the 'head-on' attack is today frequently the slowest and most expensive path to the cure and prevention of disease" (NIH Study Committee 1965: 2).

That the Woolridge-Report refers to biomedical science in the singular, however, indicates that it was not meant to be a synonym for the life sciences.[76] Furthermore, while life sciences was a concept for scientific research in the biological and medical sciences defined by a broad experimental culture, biomedical science was intended to delineate an area within this larger group that corresponded to a clear mission objective. Most importantly, therefore, the 1965 document makes clear that the NIH and the NSF were effectively responsible for funding the *same* sort of research, since the basic distinction was no longer between biology and medicine or between basic and applied sciences, but between missions. For the committee, the term acted as a means of boundary work, drawing a subtle distinction between the research sponsored under the aegis of the NIH and the NSF. The report accordingly states that the different institutes of the NIH allow for research to be assigned to potentially "all of the special disciplines that comprise the life sciences", enabling a broad coverage of research funding. And it concludes: "Thus, we may say that the primary *de facto* mission of NIH is the stimulation and support of a very broad range of health-related or biomedical research" (NIH Study Committee 1965: 3). Though talk is of the same sort of research activities, therefore, and while the idea of life sciences comprised basic research in biological and medical fields and institutions that promised to contribute to overall social progress, the NIH presented biomedical science as a broad discipline that benefitted social progress through its public health mission.

---

76 The NSF's terminology is used throughout the main text, showing that "life sciences" was also by then a normal category in the science and health policy discourse (NIH Study Committee 1965: 2, 3, 5, 7, 14, 23).

The term biomedical science has defined a disciplinary identity comprised of virtually the same research culture as that of the larger category of life sciences. The crucial difference, though, was that, in contrast to the latter, the former identity was bound to a linear legacy – the explicit promise that research in the discipline *will* lead to improvements in the nation's health.

IV. The Linear Legacy of Biomedicine

It is hard to gauge when exactly the noun biomedicine became a popular category. But by the 1980s it seems to have been widely in use. The important aspect, at least in the context of my analysis, is to consider the appearance of the noun as a manifestation of the general acceptance of the promises that are associated with the idea of basic biomedical research. In current parlance, the term biomedicine embodies the expectation that the research areas grouped under its heading will necessarily contribute to practical improvements in health care. However, removed from clinical reality, replaced in its role by clinical science and indistinguishable from the research culture of the life sciences, I argue that this feature of biomedicine is above all rhetorical.

Accounts in the sociological and historical studies of biomedicine, as already implied above, critique the idea of a linear relationship between biomedical innovation in the laboratory and their implementation in everyday clinical practice as a popular myth. Commentators have argued instead that the category describes the reality of a much more complex path to clinical innovation than is commonly captured by the post-war idea of basic research: "the existing body of scholarly work in the history of biomedicine does not support the view that laboratory research is the main (or only) source for therapeutics" (Strasser 2014: 14). For Keating and Cambrosio, the novelty of biomedicine is precisely that it "break[s] down the dichotomy" between "biomedical innovation and the translation of that innovation into a variety of medical practices" (2003: 323). Innovations in biomedicine, in other words, are the result of the collective work of scientists, clinicians, patients and other involved actors organized in relationships of a non-linear fashion – this understanding is today captured by the concept of translational research, although, authors like Keating and Cambrosio deny that the characteristic configurations of biomedicine had "to await the invention of the term 'translation research'" (ibid: 47).

The point I want to make in conclusion to this chapter is not that the scheme of the linear model adequately describes the actual processes of research, development and innovation in the medical system. I want to draw attention to the fact that the concept of biomedicine embodies such an understanding, since it was born in the climate of basic science, and that we should keep this in mind when being confronted with the expectations associated with it. Different from what some of the social studies of biomedicine claim, the promises inherent to the concept of biomedicine seem convincing not because the category transcends the linear conception underlying the ideology of basic science, but precisely because it is imbued with it. I want to illustrate some of the ideological power of the biomedical category in the current discourse by having a closer look at its semantic function.[77]

David Kaldewey has argued that despite assertions in the sociological and historical literature toward the end of the twentieth century that the so-called "linear model of innovation" was "dead", the content that the concept transports is still very much alive today (2013: 371–383). The idea of a linear model of innovation is associated less with academic than with industrial research, however. In this context, the basic understanding of the category is that the fundamental work being pursued in industrial laboratories, for instance, needs to be less abstract than academic work, to not question its future utility; it needs to be somewhat circumscribed with practical implications so that it has the possibility of offering the basis for further scientific application (ibid: 382f.).

In the current social and historical literature, as Kaldewey shows, due to a sense of crisis in science, the category has nonetheless been discarded as a viable concept in exchange for notions such as "blurring boundaries" between basic and applied research or research and development (ibid: 383). But even such conceptual renewals, which expressly distance themselves from the concept of a linear model, nevertheless transport the idea that relatively undirected basic research leads to social benefits, i.e., moves from one realm to the other (ibid: 381). A similar narrative emerged in the nineteenth century, which stated that "pure science provides the foundation for technological innovation" (Schauz 2020: 217). According to Schauz, this narrative has not lost its importance, although conceptual innovations like "technoscience" are meant as antitheses to this old understanding, standing the conceptual relationship between the natural sciences and

---

77 Keating and Cambrosio do, however, point to approaches in the second half of the twentieth century that "clearly suggested a hierarchy running from the biological to the clinical, with researchers in the latter sphere acting as applicators for knowledge produced in the former" (2004: 365).

technology on its head (ibid.). The crucial point more generally is that the semantic replacements to describe the connection of the different phases of research implied by the linear model still do not allow it to be dissociated from its underlying, century-old idea. Through "narrative means" even they postulate "a causal connection between different forms of research activities" (Kaldewey 2013: 383).

Coming from the context of the post-war basic science ideology, the concept of biomedicine precisely preserves this underlying causal notion with reference to health care – and there is public testimony to the fact that this is the central understanding of the concept. For Appel, in her account of the NSF's spending in biological fields, "the tremendous growth" of involvement of the federal government in the support of basic research in biological and related fields "vitally depended on NIH's superior ability to link research to the politically popular imperative of conquering disease" (Appel 2000: 142). Accordingly, the emergence of the category was accompanied by serious doubts about whether such a high expenditure for laboratory research could indeed deliver the promised health care benefits to the nation. In an extensive review of the Woolridge-Report in *Science*, Joseph D. Cooper, a high-ranking US government administrator and author, questions whether the health research policy of the NIH was at all structured toward any other intention than justifying large amounts of federal research spending in basic life sciences. Asking whether the agency represented a "health agency" or rather a "science agency", he concludes:

> "In short, the report [by the Woolridge Committee] states that NIH is not a disease-oriented organization. It is, rather, engaged in the support of fundamental research into life processes along normal disciplinary lines. While NIH justifies its programs to the Congress and to the public in terms of drives on various disease fronts, these are merely 'practical' expedients through which NIH has to operate" (Cooper 1965: 1435).

Critics of the NIH's spending behaviour, moreover, tend to measure the idea of biomedicine by its linear promises. In a book that elaborately and critically surveys the NIH's funding history, Edward Ahrens saw that the money being spent on basic laboratory research in the name of health care was grossly out of proportion, since its relation to clinical medicine was highly questionable:

> "The very large body of biomedical research is best described as separate from [other] categories of clinical research. These studies are performed in such varied disciplines as chemistry, physics, biology, zoolo-

gy, anatomy, biochemistry, and microbiology. While they contribute importantly to new understandings of biological processes, they are not directly related to clinical issues and do not originate in stated or implied questions dealing with human health or disease" (1992: 42).

Strictly speaking, Ahrens is critiquing the research discipline of *biomedical science*, which developed in the disputes over funding jurisdictions between the NIH and the NSF, as I just demonstrated, for making promises deriving from the supercategory of *biomedicine* – namely, as an inclusive category for a vast array of research comprising the academic health care system, which has, however, not sufficiently led to direct health care-related outcomes (Ahrens 1992). In relation, one reviewer of Ahrens' book, the American cardiologist Alvan Feinstein, even decried the category as merely a political scheme: "The hybrid term biomedicine was devised to justify the NIH's diversion, into basic molecular biology, of funds allocated for the study of human disease and health" (1995: 289).

While there can be legitimate doubt about the substance of the concept's promises, it is clear from these statements that its rhetoric worked flawlessly in convincing state officials, medical actors and the public of a linear relationship between biomedical research and the improvement of public health. An important aspect, however, is that the category could function in this way – and still does so – because of being supported by medicine's modern history. Historical events in the progress of medicine, something historian Bruno Strasser, in a recent report to the Swiss Science and Innovation Council, has termed "the collective memory of biomedicine's public successes" (2014: 13), have retrospectively undergirded the linear notion inherent in the concept of biomedicine. Among these are such famous cases as Paul Ehrlich's "magic bullet" Salvarsan, as the first cure for Syphilis (Lenoir 1997: 179–202), or the discovery of Penicillin as an antibiotic by Alexander Fleming (Bud 2007). "The rise of biomedicine," Strasser notes, "as well as its current legitimacy, owes much to the power of these stories and memories of success" (2014: 13). Thus, from society's current perspective, such (hi-)stories function as evidence for the convincing promises that the transfer of knowledge from basic research in the laboratory to the clinic will improve the reality of medical practice. But the quotes above also show how these promises have been broken in the aftermath of biomedicines ascendance. I will try to illustrate in the next chapter how actors up until now have nevertheless been able to avert a crisis of biomedicine.

7. Averting Conceptual Crisis – Semantic Stabilization of a Disciplinary Identity in the Twenty-First Century

The conceptual developments described in the previous chapter made biomedicine a broadly defined scientific discipline, which superseded the old categories of biological and medical research. But biomedicine was also bound to become a dominant and encompassing supercategory in the global science and policy discourses due to the high level of public health expectations associated with it. The term began to be understood much more broadly than only to justify the many efforts undertaken to tackle health care problems with the aid of basic research in the biosciences. Accordingly, there are references to "the biomedical research system, both basic and clinical", for example, thus indicating how biomedicine is currently the integrative concept for *all* the institutions of academic medicine (Heinig et al. 1999: 742). Similarly, in a systematic review of biomedical historiography, historian Nicolas Rasmussen understands biomedicine "as the areas of research supported and conducted by the NIH" (2018: 5). Obviously, the NIH harbors a far greater range of research types. As Edward Ahrens critically remarks: "'biomedical' is the inclusive word today for many kinds of research funded by the NIH and performed in our medical schools and medical research institutions by MDs, MD-PhDs, and others, and whose content runs the gamut from strictly biological to strictly clinical" (1992: 34).

These quotes suggest that the concept can also be viewed to comprise more than just the laboratory-based activities that I have identified as constituting the discipline. Rather, also other forms of research sponsored by the agency are subsumed under biomedicine as a supercategory – including clinical research at the bedside, which, as I showed, developed historically and institutionally distinct from the biomedical sciences. This is something to remember, when observing how biomedicine evolved into a vast research industry. The massive increase in spending for health care research and development (R&D) after World War II is a clear indication of the widespread belief in the biomedical model and its linear legacy – a belief that continues today. Additionally, a vast amount of communication on the topic has been spread through specialized publications over the past decades. A simple search for "biomed*" in publication abstracts and titles in the PubMed database, for instance, retrieves a total of 98,261 results between 1965 (the date of the Woolridge Report's publication) and 2018. Displaying these results as publications relative to all releases per year listed in the database illustrates a steady increase of output referencing biomedicine (figure 7.1).

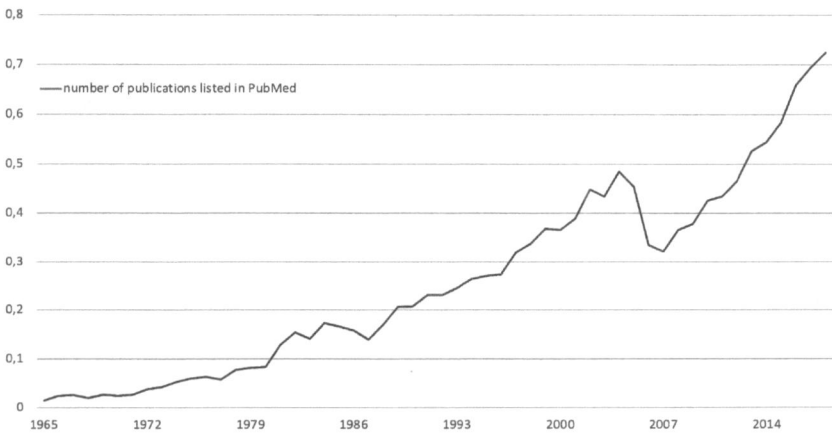

Figure 7.1:   *Graph showing relative number of publications per year with 'biomed*' in title or abstract between 1965 and 2018. (Source: PubMed database, https:// pubmed.ncbi.nlm.nih.gov/?term=%28biomed%2A%5BTitle%2FAbstract% 5D%29&filter=years.1965-2018&sort=pubdate&sort_order=asc [Accessed November 15, 2020], my visualization).*

The history of the NIH budget is also taken as an indication of the growth of the enterprise in the second half of the twentieth century. It shows a massive inflation of biomedical research and reveals the NIH to be the largest single promotor of biomedicine in the world by far (Rasmussen 2018, see also Ahrens 1992). According to the figures Rasmussen presents in his review, the NIH's budget for scientific activities grew exponentially in the decades immediately following the war. Riding on the ideological wave of basic science, he states that the "life sciences as a whole" benefitted (ibid: 8). By the late 1960s, the NIH had hit the critical mark of $1 billion in research spending. In 1970, therefore, the institute's dramatic monetary inflation dwarfed the budget of the NFS's division of Biological and Medical Sciences, which was allocated at $49 million. This highlights the "overwhelming dominance of the NIH among all US funders of life science" (ibid: 3). In that same decade, the NIH accounted for 40% of all "health R&D" expenditure in the United States, while all other government agencies combined were investing 25 %, the industry was contributing roughly 30 %, and philanthropies accounted for less than 5 % (ibid., see also Ahrens 1992: 65–79). Although the budget of the agency plateaued in this period, funds for biomedical science began to increase again in the mid-1980s as the Cold War reached its second peak (ibid: 9). Today, the NIH continues to be the largest single funder in the field globally.[78] As stated on its homepage, the agency invests "about \$41,7 billion annually in medical research for the American people".[79] Only in the mid-2000s, did the share of world health research and development conducted publicly by the United States fall beneath 50 %, although public and private spending combined at the time still accounted for more than half of the expenditure worldwide (ibid: 3).

That biomedicine had also become an accepted scientific discipline, however, can be taken from the imprints bearing its name. As I showed in the first chapters of my book, medical actors in the past used the founding of academic journals to arrange the medical discipline according to their ideals and interests. Journals can thus act as an indicator of how disciplines become integrated into the academic landscape since they represent a format through which actors within a scientific community communicate with each other and accordingly contribute to the growth of their field (Stichweh 2007). In wake of the recategorization from scientific medicine into biomedicine in the 1960s, specialized journals began appearing and contributed to the constitution of a biomedical discipline. It would require an extensive content analysis to see which of these journals represent the discipline genuinely and which have adopted the vocabulary more out of rhetorical reasons to connect themselves to the vastly growing biomedical enterprise under the supercategory – something that is beyond the scope of my investigation, though. Nevertheless, if we search the database Web of Science for publications in journals with "biomed*" in the title, it retrieves a total of 56,769 items between 1971 and 2019 (there appears to be no significant output before that timespan). The 1970s, moreover, appear to have been a critical time for establishing biomedical journals, launching at least four new journals bearing the category in its title (table 7.2).

---

78 In comparison to the NIH, the German Ministry of Education and Research (BMBF) spent more than 2.6 billion of its total 23 billion Euro research-budget on health-related investigations in 2017, with an increase of roughly 400 million Euros in budget and 100 million Euros in medical research spending in 2018. These figures were taken from the 2018 BMBF-report: https://www.bmbf.de/pub/Bufi_2018_Datenband.pdf (accesses August 20, 2020).

79 https://www.nih.gov/about-nih/what-we-do/budget (accessed August 20, 2020).

The ambiguity of biomedicine as a scientific discipline and a supercategory that exhibits the ability to subsume vast areas of heterogeneous activities in medicine has caused serious tensions between different actors in the academic system. Particularly practitioners in clinical fields soon began to perceive that the massive investments made in the name of biomedicine were unjustified. Especially molecular biology, with its stellar ascent in international science, was causing significant frictions. This "new biology" had evolved into a dominant discipline by the 1950s, coming from the collective work of chemists, physicists and biologists. The field emerged from studies relating to human physiology and pathology and was therefore present in many American medical schools, but it quickly transcended any immediate relevance to these areas (Kohler 1982: 324ff.). Nonetheless, its paradigm was seen to significantly relocate the study of processes of life and disease to the level of molecules, which could be investigated using microorganisms as models as well as with the aid of more and more sophisticated analytical techniques (Kay 1993, see also Rheinberger 2009).

first issue	journal title	ISSN
1967	*Journal of Biomedical Materials Research*	0021-9304
1970	*International Journal of Biomedical Computing*	1136-5056
1971*	*Biomedical Engineering / Biomedizinische Technik*	0013-5585
1972	*Annals of Biomedical Engineering*	0090-6964
1973	*Biomedicine: The European Journal of Clinical and Biological Research*	0300-0893
	Biomédicine la Revue Européenne d'Études Cliniques et Biologiques	
1982*	*Biomedicine & Pharmacoptherapie / Biomédicine & Pharmacothérapie*	0753-3322
2001	*Journal of Biomedicine and Biotechnology*	1110-7251

Table 7.2: A selection of journals published since the 1960s bearing 'biomedical' or 'biomedicine' in the title. Asterisk (*) indicates that the journal was founded earlier but under a different name.

Molecular biology therefore implied that it was possible to study disease removed from the clinic and the patient, which made practical expertise in clinical medicine virtually obsolete.[80] The way molecular biology was performing "engendered a trend in which those undertaking research into disease were drawn increasingly to the laboratory bench" (Kraft 2013:

---

80 With respect to the "crisis" in clinical research see also the 2004 special issue of *Perspectives in Biology and Medicine* (Schechter/Perlman/Retting 2004).

28). As molecular biology research communities boarded the biomedical bandwagon, the field was receiving an ever-increasing share of funds from health care R&D-budgets, especially from the NIH, which acted as one of the major supporters of molecular biology during the Cold War Era (Appel 2000: 209–216). As a result, renown departments with apparently no clinical connection were built using NIH funds, like the "molecular biology hothouse" in Stanford University's biochemistry department (in the medical school!), "where luminaries like Paul Berg and Arthur Kornberg solved the riddles of gene expression in *E. coli* bacteria" (Rasmussen 2018: 6).

Molecular biology has strongly influenced the public image of what it means to do research in medicine after World War II (Strasser 2014: 12). But the dominant picture of molecular biology also entailed a superimposition of its cultural understanding onto the culture of clinical science. As is apparent throughout my book, medical scientists in preclinical as well as clinical departments have generally been physicians by training (even if they often refrained from any form of medical practice). While clinical departments remained dominated (and controlled) by medical doctors, the professional composition in preclinical departments began to change as sciences such as physiology or biochemistry started awarding their own graduate degrees by the start of the twentieth century. In 1992, Ahrens saw that also "the focus of clinical investigators" had "shifted dramatically" since the 1960s, from patient-oriented clinical research towards *in vivo* studies of disease using animal models and *in vitro* studies of human materials such as blood or tissue. He attributed this development to "a fascination with the power of the new reductionist technologies of molecular biology to reach new insights at the molecular level and to do so rapidly" (1992: 48).

At the same time, however, the conceptual contours of what it meant to do work in clinical science had themselves become critically unclear. In a 1999 review of clinical research in the United States, the authors detected that the collection of reliable data was hampered by a "wide discrepancy in the *definitions of clinical research*" and that the lack of a universally accepted definition "led to variability and contentiousness in accepting the designation of different kinds of research activities as 'clinical'" (Heinig et al. 1999: 727, see also Schechter/Perlman/Rettig 2004: 479f.). As I illustrated in chapter 5, clinical science evolved at the start of the twentieth century when actors adopted the scientific ideology of laboratory work but directed its methods to issues of clinical practice. In a current definition, therefore, "clinical investigations may encompass the whole gamut of research activities, including analyses of disease pathophysiology (for which sophisticated study of normal human biochemistry and physiology is necessary); of the prevention, cause, and course of disease; and of the effects of interventions (pharmacologic, surgical, behavioral, etc.) on human health" (Schechter/Perlman/Rettig 2004: 480).

Consequently, the activity describes an integrative approach to the study of disease in patients. This form of scientific activity, "synonymous with 'experimental medicine', 'clinical science', and 'clinical investigation'" (Ahrens 1992: 39), is aided by consultations with a clinical laboratory, but not reduced to it. Clinical science requires both proficiency in clinical care *and* basic research.

However, torn between the bedside and the bench, and subject to attempts in the early decades of the twentieth century to also widen the idea of clinical science towards population-based inquiries, it had become unclear what clinical science's methods and approaches to study the treatment of disease precisely entailed. Not the least has this ambiguity been accelerated by the overall success of molecular research under the wings of the supercategory biomedicine. According to historian Alison Kraft, clinical research constituted "a slippery term" by the end of the twentieth century, associated with a range of activities, "from patient-centered research at the bedside, to lab-based research into the molecular basis of disease, to the clinical trial" (2013: 33f., see also Borck 2020: 459). Accordingly, witnessing an increase in the numbers of non-medical doctors in clinical departments since the 1970s, Ahrens warned his readers that it would be a mistake to consider postdoctoral scientists "in clinical departments merely as individuals hired to perform laboratory work", which medical doctors have increasingly little time for, "or simply as supervisors of technicians in those laboratories" (1992: 25). Rather, the development indicated a colonization of clinical institutions by researchers in fields of the basic sciences. With biomedicine designating the whole complex of academic medicine and the concept of clinical science also comprising activities of basic laboratory research, therefore, the outlines of what were once deemed preclinical and clinical domains had faded. This induced a stronger reliance on the linear promises in the public understanding of biomedicine, while it also entailed a differentiation of the professional functions of actors in clinical medicine. An increasing divide between the practice of clinical medicine and clinical investigation on the one side and the research function of medical science was emerging in the institution, "and whilst some clinicians continued with clinical investigation in the patient at the bedside, many others pursued a different kind of clinical research in the laboratory" (Kraft 2013: 30, see also Ahrens 1992: 48).

What were the consequences of such conceptual and professional ambiguities? And how did actors try to avert the looming crisis in medical research and clinical care? The shifting conceptions over roles and functions in the academic health care system meant that the idea of the physician as a scientific investigator in the historical sense was on the wane. At the same time, in its supercategorical dimension, biomedicine was assuming more direct responsibility for improvements in clinical medicine than its scientific discipline originally promised. This required clarifications, conceptually and institutionally, of what the relationship between the biomedical discipline and the system of clinical medicine comprised. I want to use this chapter to look at two recent categories that have not altered the meaning of biomedicine as such, but which have stabilized its general understanding by redefining the institutional structures of academic medicine with respect to clinical practice and research – evidence-based medicine (EBM) and translational research (TR). These categories emerged at the end of the twentieth and the start of the twenty-first century, respectively. If viewed from the perspective of conceptual and institutional history, they appear to have somewhat of an entangled semantic function. I argue that they work to recategorize the different areas of medical science by clarifying the position of clinical research and practice in face of the dominating biomedical concept.

On the one side, EBM corresponds mainly to biomedicine as a scientific discipline and acts to confirm its autonomy vis-à-vis clinical medicine. The concept is carried by a deep-seated dissatisfaction with the paradigm that bases practical medicine on explanations in knowledge of the biomedical laboratory. It therefore transitions the cultural foundation of clinical practice away from the lab to population-based reasoning and through the institutionalization of clinical guidelines. TR, on the other side, correspond to biomedicine as a supercategory and the vast research enterprise it harbors. The concept reinforces the idea of biomedicine's linear legacy by integrating into it a reinvented version of the historical ideal of the physician-researcher. This category, in other words, confirms the autonomy of the biomedical discipline through institutional distinction. But it also preserves its identity by confirming the linear legacy, connecting biomedicine semantically to the vague category of "clinical science".

I. Evidence-Based Medicine and the New Cultural Foundation of Clinical Practice

The debate about evidence-based medicine (EBM) is too vast and still ongoing as that it could be reasonably summarized here (see e.g., Cohen et al. 2004, Daly 2005: 102–127, 206–234, Knaapen 2014, Solomon 2011, also Borck 2020, Weisz 2005). Hence, I only want to show how the category was defined at its inception and point to its semantic function regarding the understanding of the relationship between biomedicine and clinical medicine. The main purpose of the category, in this respect, is to semantically remove practical medicine from a cultural foundation in the biomedical discipline, while maintaining a strictly scientific foundation for medical practice. Although EBM ostensibly brings a standardization to the practice of health care (Knaapen 2014, Timmermans/Berg 2003), the category can, in a sense, also be seen as the successful founding of clinical medicine on epidemiological instead of biomedical premises (Daly 2005).

I want to argue that this change of practical foundation confirmed the status of biomedicine as an autonomous discipline within the larger academic complex. Epidemiology had developed from an observation-based and dismissively treated approach for public health officials in the early decades of the twentieth century into a genuine scientific discipline in the post-war era. It incorporated the "experimental ideal" but transferred it to the study of disease in populations using statistical methods, thereby elevating itself to the same level scientifically as the laboratory sciences (Amsterdamska 2005). Epidemiology thus constituted an apt candidate for relocating practical medicine to a scientifically sound foundation, especially in an age that was anyhow increasingly adhering to the apparent soundness of statistical inference (Borck 2020: 455ff.).

Since about the 1960s, actors were making efforts to find ways to ensure that care was being delivered to patients according to clearly discernible and reproducible premises (as opposed to physicians' intuition or routine). The emergence of the discipline of clinical epidemiology in Canada and the United States at the time manifested this motivation to bring the population-based approaches characteristic of public health studies also to clinical medicine. Through its focus on quantitative methods for investigating clinical practice empirically, "clinical epidemiology represented a new way of thinking about clinical care that its proponents described as representing a paradigm shift" (Daly 2005: 4). Reminiscent of the developments in clinical science, which were illustrated in chapter 5, actors were framing the discipline as a new "basic science for clinical medicine" (Borck 2020: 461).

Obviously, it was a difficult venture to simply shift the deeply rooted knowledge base of medical practice to the discipline of clinical epidemiology and its culture of statistical reasoning, given the historical tradition of socializing physicians in the habits of the laboratory sciences. A group of epidemiologists and clinicians from Canada and the United States formed the core of advocates for the new key medical concept of EBM. In 1992, they boldly proclaimed the advent of "A NEW paradigm for medical practice", in an article in the *Journal of the American Medical Association* that acts as the founding document for the movement:

> "Evidence-based medicine de-emphasizes intuition, unsystematic clinical experience, and pathophysiologic rationale as sufficient grounds for clinical decision making and stresses the examination of evidence from clinical research. Evidence-based medicine requires new skills of the physician, including efficient literature searching and the application of formal rules of evidence evaluating the clinical literature." (EBM Working Group 1992: 2420)

The proclaimed novelty of the movement deferred the attention away from the fact that, historically, clinical medicine and public health, from which the methods derived, were in fact institutionally divided. Very generally speaking, clinicians dealt with individual patients and their diseases, while public health had a far broader scope incorporating many perspectives onto the everyday lives of people and their relation to health. This division was of course a source of friction (Daly 2005: 121ff.).

The group of epidemiologists and clinicians promoting EBM therefore introduced it as "A New Approach to Teaching and the Practice of Medicine" (EBM Working Group 1992: 2420). Instead of merely transferring medical practice to an epidemiological basis, they thereby simply justified the change on the grounds of inserting new pedagogical ideals into medical practice, which nonetheless focused on statistical and epidemiological methods, including systematic ways to appraise the professional literature (Borck 2020: 462ff., Daly 2005: 75ff.). According to David Sackett, a leading proponent and practitioner of EBM, and his colleagues, the approach was defined as "the conscientious, explicit, and judicious use of current best evidence in making decisions about the care of individual patients" (Sackett et al. 1996: 71). This meant that medical treatments were to be investigated in population-based clinical studies to generate such evidence for medical care, particularly using randomized controlled trials

(RCTs), which had emerged as the "gold standard" for evaluating drug safety and efficacy in the United States (Marks 1997). RCTs constituted a relatively simple but powerful transfer of the experimental design characteristic of investigations in the natural sciences to the study of clinical populations. "Its promise was that it would achieve the rigor, and certainty, of laboratory findings" (Daly 2005: 13). Together with the technique of meta-analysis, a way of statistically aggregating the results of various clinical studies of the same intervention, these methods were meant to continually update the "objective" basis for clinical care by invalidating "previously accepted diagnostic tests and treatments" and replacing them "with new ones that are more powerful, more accurate, more efficacious, and safer" (Sackett et al. 1996: 71).

Historian of medicine Cornelius Borck convincingly demonstrates how the category of EBM entailed a reorganization of the epistemic hierarchy governing clinical medicine. Not only did its advocates discard the "three historically most important ways of legitimising medicine" (i.e. as an art, an expertise and a science) (Borck 2020: 463); in their program, "theoretical knowledge and scientific explanations were downgraded epistemologically, from previously ranking as the highest form of knowledge in biomedicine to now functioning as a mere heuristic or useful strategy for identifying possible targets for new interventions (then to be evaluated by RCTs)" (ibid: 464). As with the case of emphasizing the scientific methodology in the medical curriculum to downgrade the epistemological place of clinical medicine in mid-nineteenth century Germany, in other words, the concept of EBM effectively meant that the foundation of the clinician's professional culture transitioned from being grounded foremost on experimental laboratory methods to epidemiological techniques.

According to this new ideology, knowledge of pathophysiology was still required but it was now also regarded as insufficient for practicing clinical medicine. "All pathophysiological inferences should be subordinated to the question of whether diagnostic or therapeutic interventions have been proven to be effective in sound empirical studies" (Timmermans/Kolker 2004: 183). While professional training of physicians still remains dominated by laboratory sciences, areas that proponents of EMB favored have also made it into today's curriculum. At the University of Bonn, for instance, students of medicine are required to take courses in "medical statistics", "epidemiology, biometry, and informatics", and "medical informatics", next to courses in pathology, clinical chemistry, and other medical topics, in their first clinical semester (the fifth semester overall).[81] The original intention of the EBM movement was indeed to train doctors in the critical appraisal of the literature, that is, precisely in such fields. The idea was that clinicians should always be up to date with respect to the statistics of which treatments best applied to what cases. But this original ideal largely failed due to practical reasons: it conflicted with the busy workload of practicing clinicians. So, in contrast to the nineteenth century, where protagonists altered the cultural basis of medicine through changes in the curriculum, EBM has ended up changing the professional culture less through the explicit exposure to epidemiology at the student level, than through the introduction of guidelines into everyday clinical practice, which can be composed relatively easily based on meta-analytic studies (Weisz et al. 2007: 713).

II. Shifting the Basis of Clinical Medicine Through Guidelines

It is not my intention to go into any detail about the historical developments leading to the emergence of clinical guidelines (see Weisz et al. 2007); nor to engage in debates about the role of guidelines for the undermining or preserving of physicians' professional autonomy (Armstrong 2007, Timmermans/Kolker 2004, Vogd 2002). All I want to do here is shed a light on functional aspects of the category that serve the purpose of sustaining the argument that the biomedical discipline no longer constitutes the cultural foundation of practical medicine. But how can guidelines be seen as an indication of biomedicine's institutional autonomy?

Clinical guidelines have been presented as changing the way that the quality of medical practice is controlled. "Until the 1970s," according to George Weisz and his collaborators, "medical actions were indirectly regulated through the training and credentials guaranteed by both the organized profession and state authorities" (Weisz et al. 2007: 693). In the context of my elaboration, in other words, the quality of medical practices was guaranteed by the professional culture in which physicians were socialized during their studies. Self-governing bodies like medical associations made sure that the study courses providing the socialization upheld the required standards of medical practice. With the increasing

---

81 See the relevant information on the medical faculty's website: https://www.medfa k.uni-bonn.de/de/lehre-studium/studiengaenge/humanmedizin/klinik/daten-und -plaene (accessed 15. November 2020).

importance of clinical guidelines since about the 1980s, however, this measure of control has been externalized from physicians, their experience and knowledge of pathophysiological processes to *"procedural standards that specify the actions or protocols that must be followed in given situations"* (ibid.).[82] The making of these standards, in turn, can be explained as a process of negotiated conventions, something Keating, Cambrosio and colleagues have conceptualized as "regulatory objectivity" (Cambrosio et al. 2006). A closer look at the idea of regulatory objectivity in the context of guidelines, which draws on the authors' preliminary work about biomedical platforms, will help answer this question.

The idea of regulatory objectivity describes a recursive procedure by which conventions guiding clinical practices are coordinated with those guiding the research process. In contrast to the concepts of objectivity of former times, the authors argue, "regulatory objectivity turns the focus away from objects towards collective forms of expertise combining people (clinicians, researchers, administrators, patients, etc.) and objects (entities, instruments, tools, techniques, etc.) connected by specific coordination regimes" (ibid: 194, see also Keating/Cambrosio 2012: 20f., 25ff.). The crucial point for my argument is that in the coordinated regime of RCTs, which lies at the heart of EBM, the correlation between the conventions of biomedical knowledge production and clinical action have been supplanted by that of the narrower focus of producing knowledge of effective interventions in the clinic. In face of this development, the EBM movement, as I explained, required that clinicians abandon intuition, clinical experience and pathophysiologic rationale and instead demanded that "evaluation be based on distinctions among levels of evidence" (Weisz et al. 2007: 713). Effectively, this meant a rejection of the confidence that scientific explanations can justify therapeutic interventions. Borck puts it most clearly, when he summarizes that, according to the fundamentals of EBM, "evidence suffices even in the absence of explanations, something which is absolutely unsatisfactory for science-based medicine" (2020: 466).

EBM thus infuses the basis of clinical practice with the priority for an epidemiological and not a biomedical understanding. An intervention

---

82 Reasons given for this development are "the increasing role of governments in every aspect of health care" and "the perceived need in nearly all Western nations to impose rational direction and coordination on an array of [health care] institutions [...] that had been created incrementally and almost haphazardly over long periods of time that were increasing both in size and technological-functional complexity." (Weisz et al. 2007: 704f.).

is deemed legitimate not if the science says that it works, but if it has statistically been proven to work and if this "proof" is enshrined in clinical guidelines for best practice. Since RCTs form the single most important procedure for producing viable clinical evidence and meta-analysis is, in turn, the effective basis to produce guidelines: the actions of clinicians are no longer regulated primarily by biomedical explanations but by the coordinated conventions of population-based methods and clinical practice. In short, the introduction of EBM into academic discourses represents the climax of the differentiation between biomedical science and clinical care, which started in the Progressive Era. This does not mean that biomedicine and the clinic have nothing to do with each other anymore – far from it. But it does entail the fundamental restructuring of the epistemic hierarchies and research cultures that lay the foundations for medical practice. Like Virchow's program of scientific medicine, which moved the science of experimental physiology in the background to henceforth constitute the general framework in which medical science was performed, so, too, EBM has delegated biomedical science to constitute the general context in which clinical care is researched. But through the instruments of EBM, the conceptual basis for medical practice shifted away from the requirement of biomedical knowledge. In this constellation, clinical medicine has not only found a new scientific basis; EBM furthermore confirms the position of biomedicine as a discipline distinct from clinical responsibilities. Therefore, it stabilizes the original meaning of biomedical science – the post-war era basic research cultures in biology and medicine that hold the possibility to improve public health but cannot be pressed too hard on delivering that promise.

III. Confirming the Linear Legacy with Translational Science

If EBM targeted the concept of clinical practice, TR can be said to aim at reorganizing the idea of clinical science in the twenty-first century, especially in the wake of molecular biology and genetics. However, since EBM acts to confirm biomedicine in its remote contributions to the betterment of public health, TR offers a semantic correction that reinforces the linear legacy of the bench-bedside-connection. EBM functioned to differentiate clinical medicine from biomedicine by introducing its version of "clinical science", based on epidemiological reasoning, and removed from laboratory culture. TR also references "clinical science", however, framing it as an integral part of biomedicine to suggest its continued relevance for health care. TR is also a concept that has received its deserved share of sociological investigations and the research landscape is increasing steadily (see Crabu 2018, also Mittra/Milne 2013). The purpose here is therefore again to only examine the category for its functional aspects in the current science and policy discourses with respect to the idea of biomedicine and the culture of clinical research.

The way the term TR is used can be distinguished roughly into a broader dimension, addressing a supposed breach in the biomedical innovation pipeline on the one side, and aiming more concretely at bridging the gap between basic research at the bench and patient treatment in the clinic on the other. Both meanings are interrelated, although commentators tend to find their underlying rationales to be contradictory. In most cases, TR is associated with the idea of a linear model of innovation or a continuum leading from the laboratory bench to clinical application. The implication is that the knowledge generated through basic biomedical research is meant to be translated into "ideas and knowledge about real (diseased) bodies and in[to] medical technologies", which then seek implementation in practical medicine (van der Laan/Boenink 2015: 39). The prevalence of this idea can be attributed to the ideological power of basic science, which in the case of biomedicine has been fueled by the dominance of molecular biology, leading to "an interpretation of the dynamic between the lab and the clinic as one in which, predominantly, information flowed from bench to bedside", as Kraft observes (2013: 29). Nonetheless, commentators on TR point out that the view of biomedical R&D as a linear and largely one-directional innovation process is "empirically inadequate" (van der Laan/Boenink 2015: 40f.) or "rarely reflects the reality on the ground" (Mittra 2016: 60).

My aim is not to prove or disprove the adequacy of the idea of a continuum between bench and bedside; just like I did not want to assess, in the conclusion to chapter 6, any kind of correspondence between the linearity engrained into the category of biomedicine and the empirical reality of biomedical research. Instead, I want to show how the underlying narrative of linearity was appropriated by protagonists in clinical science to stake out their professional turf by framing it as translation work regarding both spheres. Sociologists investigating the TR concept have shown that, as these clinician-scientists faced increasing incursions into their domain from pure laboratory-based research, the professional hierarchy within the biomedical system tilted to their disadvantage (Wilson-Kovacz/Hauskeller 2012, see also Mittra 2016: 96f.). To push back against the expanding boundary of the biomedical discipline, these actors aligned themselves with other actors in the research policy front at the start of the twenty-first century, contributing to the formulation of the institutional requirements to pursue their professional interests (Vignola-Gagné 2014). Thus, rather than seeing the two understandings of the relation between laboratory and clinic enshrined into the category of TR as contradictory, we can regard it as a rhetorical strategy, in which both meanings are directed at two different discourses. These discourses emerged subsequently and relate to the professional culture of the clinician-scientist and health care R&D, respectively. More, we can observe that "translational research" was a prevalent category in the English-speaking world before "translational science" and "translational medicine" became important denotations (figure 7.3). As in the case of biomedicine, this indicates that we first had the description of the practices before they became used as a mark to distinguish a specific scientific culture, which was afterwards institutionalized in the academic system.

IV. The Character of Translation Practices

The term TR first emerged in the early 1990s in the field of cancer research, where it was associated with a bi-directional understanding of linking basic and clinical science but quickly spread to other biomedical fields after 2000 (van der Laan/Boenik 2015: 34f., see also Keating/Cambrosio 2012: 348). The meaning of TR "slightly shifted" after 2003, according to Anna Laura van der Laan and Marianne Boenink in a review of TR in the literature, from a "desire to finally see effective treatment for an awful disease [cancer]" to the assessment "that health improvements have not kept up with the increased speed of discovery in the life sciences", particularly in fields like genomics and molecular biology (2015: 36). In that year, the newly elected head of the NIH, Elias Zerhouni, initiated "The Roadmap" mentioned in the introduction, which aimed at reforming key processes of the institutes' biomedical R&D along the lines of three major themes – "New Pathways to Discovery, Research Teams of the Future, and Reengineering the Clinical Research Enterprise" (2003: 63). The policies of the NIH Roadmap were meant to address "today's pressing scientific challenges" and "roadblocks to progress" brought on especially through the sequencing of the human genome; they were intended to adapt the activities conducted under the agency's aegis to concomitant redefinitions of "the ways that medical research is conducted and, ultimately, how research leads to improvements in health" (ibid). Zerhouni – himself a clinician-scientist from Johns Hopkins' department of radiological science – argued for the necessity of major organizational and infrastructural changes in order to facilitate that discoveries in the laboratory made it into clinical innovations, whereby TR was to constitute itself as "the new paradigm in biomedical research" (Kraft 2013: 43).

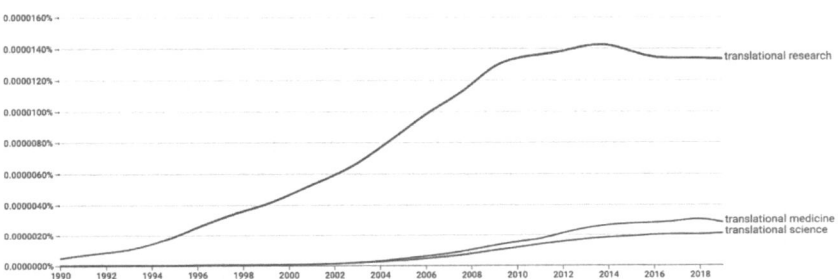

Figure 7.3:   Word frequencies of "translational research", "translational medicine" and "translational science", 1990–2019. (Source: Google Books Ngram Viewer, https://books.google.com/ngrams/graph?year=_end=2019&year_start=1990& content=translational+research%2Ctranslational+science%2Ctranslational+ medicine&smoothing=3&corpus=26 [accessed September 1, 2020]).

Zerhouni's Roadmap can be regarded as the political strategy that connects the interests of a R&D innovation system understanding itself in linear terms with those of the clinician-scientists, who see themselves straddling at the interface of the laboratory and the clinic. It inspired an era in which more and more policies for TR were implemented in different countries that began to justify the role of the clinician-scientist as an important element in health care innovation (Hendriks/Simon/Reinhart 2019: 227, Kraft 2013: 45f., Mittra 2016: 71ff.). Empirical studies point to how the actual work of clinician scientists "is overburdened with vague or completely unspecified expectations" regarding the task of translating research (ibid: 233). This has to do mostly with the fact that these actors need to operate simultaneously as caregivers in the clinic and as bench researchers. Not only are both activities inherently time consuming, the increasing specialization in biomedical science also makes it nearly impossible to keep up for someone who is not devoted to the field full-time.

I want to nevertheless try and identify professional markers of the clinician-scientist circulating in the discourses of TR, so that it becomes clear how their scientific culture was distinguished from that of the biomedical discipline and from earlier understandings of clinical research. In this regard, Kraft succinctly notes that the meaning of the term TR is at the same time vague, comprising a range of activities, actors and sectors part of the biomedical enterprise, and also "highly specific, in that in practice it is defined differently by different actors [...] in ways that reflect their position within the innovation process" (2013: 46). The long-standing ambiguities in the meaning of clinical science, which I discussed above, made it necessary for its principal actors to redefine their work in a way that would distinguish it from that of the basic researcher. Describing their activities in terms of the vague concept of TR allowed them to be characterized in the new guise of the clinician-scientist and put them at the forefront of the biomedical system in the twenty-first century.

Forming the basis of the Roadmap programs was "an ethos supportive of the view that clinical insight had a role to play in shaping 'basic' research" (ibid: 43). This was a reaction to the overgrown role that basic research, especially in molecular biology, was playing in the fight against disease. Accordingly, a central requirement for any clinician-scientist is "to be able to speak the two languages of research and clinic" (Hendriks/Simon/Reinhart 2019: 233). As a result, in the case of stem cell research, for example, they describe their role as treating patients and contributing to the biological understanding of disease (Wilson-Kovacz/Hauskeller 2015: 501). These are not equal concerns, however. Understanding mechanisms is presented as only secondary to the actual aim of improving patient health (ibid: 503).

In this respect, the clinician-scientist of the translational era differs little from the clinical scientist that emerged as an actor at the start of the twentieth century and who was proficient enough in lab work to aid his/her investigations in the clinic with the aid of the natural sciences (see Harvey 1981). But with the increasing specialization in science and medicine, the clinical researcher taking an integrated pathophysiological approach to the study of disease appeared outdated in a world in which the way that medical research was conducted had become redefined into constituting specialties targeting very specific areas of the human metabolism (Hendriks/Simon/Reinhart 2019: 230). A crucial innovation, therefore, was to make the culture of clinical trials in different configurations a distinguishing feature of the clinician-scientist in the TR discourses.[83] However, trials were no longer aimed mainly at assessing the efficacy and safety of new therapeutics, as they conventionally did, but to answer

---

83 The Roadmap included a significant push for, in the long run, associating clinical research with the trial (Kraft 2013: 42).

specific research questions pertaining to the functioning of the human body and its responses to deliberate interventions. Moreover, the practice of clinical trials for research purposes endowed the clinician-scientist with an aura of clinical medicine. Thus, it confirmed the relationship between biomedicine and the clinic.

In their study of clinician-scientists in stem cell research, sociologists Dana Wilson-Kovacz and Christine Hauskeller argue that the RCT plays a central role for the scientific culture of TR in stem cell science. They show that such trials "are orchestrated by a distinct type of medical professional who devotes time to biological research and clinical practice", who accordingly incorporates proficiencies of basic and applied science, and therefore presents himself/herself as in possession of "the right skills to translate this knowledge into potential therapies" (2012: 507). The adoption of this form of practice as a professional mark of the clinician-scientist can be traced to the practice of oncology, where the concept of TR first emerged.

In their second major contribution to the social and historical study of science and medicine in the post-war world, *Cancer on Trial*, Keating and Cambrosio, based on a rich historiography of central political, organizational and epistemic moments of clinical oncology in Europe and the United States, demonstrate how since the 1950s clinical trials were developing into their own style of doing biomedical research. Although the authors dismiss the category of TR as a "catchphrase" and as "but the most recent organizational expression of the ongoing molecular biology turn" (Keating/Cambrosio 2012: 348f.), their book nonetheless provides a valuable analytical angle to understand clinical trials as a distinct professional culture defining the jurisdiction of the clinician-scientist in the era of TR. While clinical trials traditionally function to assess the performance of treatments, Keating and Cambrosio argue that in oncology "clinical trials have become full-fledged experiments" (ibid: 21). They have contributed to the generation of "a whole new class of sui generis objects that, in turn, have redefined the practices of clinicians, statisticians, and biologists" and thus constitute a system, which "contains its own reflexive machinery for establishing facts as well as how those facts should be integrated into evolving networks of concepts" (ibid: 21f.).

For Wilson-Kovacs and Hauskeller, moreover, the clinical trial not only represents "an essential step in producing an independent, autonomous and self-contained area of knowledge", it also is a resource for clinician-scientists to "reinforce their key position at the intersection between traditional medical care, scientific research and academic medicine" (2012: 507f.). What distinguishes the research culture of clinical trials in oncology, according to Keating and Cambrosio, is its reorientation towards molecular biology (2012: 350ff.). Initially, oncological research was devoted to the classification of cancerous disease in living human subjects. In the context of conducting molecular cancer clinical trials, the adjacent studies "differed from previous laboratory studies by shifting the emphasis from natural history to mechanisms" (ibid: 352). One way to orient the practice of clinical trials within this new regime is, for instance, by integrating biomarkers into the study protocol.

Biomarkers are indicators, which allow the measurement of biological processes or conditions. They hold somewhat of a prominent position within the discourses of TR, since they can link clinical values such as symptoms to detectible bodily processes (Mittra 2016: 80f.). In the context of clinical trials, therefore, biomarkers often function as "surrogate endpoints" as opposed to the traditional clinical endpoints (van der Laan/ Boenink 2015: 43, see also Keating/Cambrosio 2012: 367). This means that the outcome of an investigation is no longer if a certain intervention has an effect on a specific condition, but on how it alters and changes bodily processes. The innovation of conducting trials with biomarker endpoints thus lies in the targeted approach, which they enable. It now becomes possible to investigate the correlation of an administered compound to a specific biological process or condition, instead of asking – as in the case of traditional RCTs – how a treatment behaves overall in a certain population (Keating/Cambrosio 2012: 361). The clinical trial of TR thus requires of its practitioners no longer simply clinical and epidemiological skills, but also knowledge of molecular mechanisms – a combination embodied only in the new figure of the clinician-scientist. The University of Bonn accordingly offers physicians inclined to do research in translational medicine the possibility of a three-year scholarship program to become "clinician-scientists" after they have completed their residency. The aim of the course is to, in "cooperation between the clinics and the basic-oriented research groups as well as the theoretical institutes", provide fellows with enough flexibility to pursue their own projects, next to their clinical duties.[84] In a sense, therefore, TR constitutes a program to structurally reinforce the institution of clinical science in a time when academic medicine is dominated by research in molecular biology.

---

84 See the description on the medical faculty's homepage: https://www.medfak.uni -bonn.de/de/qualifikation-karriere/karriere/karrierewege-und-ausbildung-201eclin ician-scientist201c (accessed November 15, 2020).

For Keating and Cambrosio clinical trials in oncology simply constitute a new style of biomedical practice. With Becher and Trowler we could better say that trials in TR show how the academic tribe of clinical science settled on a new territory of biological research. It transformed a method originally designed for the assessment of best evidence for clinical practice into a new scientific tool for drug research. Taken together, we can thus see how the categories of EBM and TR in the current discourse on biomedicine function to confirm the autonomy of the biomedical discipline while at the same time reinforcing the linear legacy it transports, especially regarding the supercategory. This becomes possible because both categories insert ideas of clinical medicine and clinical science into the academic and research policy discourse that have somewhat conflicting meanings and functions. EBM constitutes an emancipation of both biomedicine and clinical medicine from each other by shifting the cultural foundation of clinical practice from biomedical to epidemiological reasoning. This enables biomedicine *qua* biomedical science to continue as an independent academic discipline next to disciplines like physics, chemistry or biology.

TR, in a sense, appropriates the new clinical science culture for biomedicine to, beyond the structural independence of the biomedical discipline, affirm a connection of the vast and heterogenous research field to public health matters. Any basic lab research can now be seen in this light if it adheres to categories like biomarkers. Thus, institutionalization of TR in clinical science and medicine also reinforces the linear legacy in the biomedical supercategory that integrates the various scientific and clinical practices, which make up academic medicine and a large part of research in the biosciences today. While clinician-scientists describe their work in different terms, by framing it as part of TR, the idea of translation itself, "coupled with the rhetoric of a broken R&D system," suggests the existence of a "linear health innovation pathway" and the continuity of a distinction between basic and applied research (Mittra 2016: 59). What is interesting about this constellation, is that TR also affirms the relative distance that biomedicine as a discipline has to improvements in clinical medicine. By introducing a new culture of clinical science, it works similar to the introduction of clinical medicine as a pure science at the start of the twentieth century – wedging a new discipline into the relationship between sciences of the laboratory and the clinic, thereby removing the former from responsibility for the latter.

8. Conclusion – Biomedicine as Discipline and Integrational Category

In my book, I set out to recover the lost disciplinary identity of medicine. In the process, I tried to give historical explanations of the complicated relationships between institutions like the laboratory, the clinic, the natural, the medical and the clinical sciences as well as medical practice. In short, I wanted to provide a historical picture of academic medicine from the vantage point of *scientific*, rather than clinical practice. I was able to show that medicine is more than just a science-based profession; that it rather constitutes an autonomous academic discipline, next to others like physics, chemistry or biology. For this purpose, it was important to realize that reference to an epistemic object or a shared set of practices is only one aspect of a scientific discipline. The theoretical approach of disciplinary cultures helped me elucidate this fact. The concept constitutes sort of a middle ground between sociological notions of disciplinarity and the idea of research cultures popular in STS. It is meant to go beyond the formal understanding of disciplines, defined by such features as paradigms, canons, recruitment structures or the institutionalization in departments; and complement it with a perspective on the more individual and local conditions in which disciplines are formed and changed.

Although the structures defining the scientific system have been shown to be not as orderly as the sociologies of science suggest, my study presents a strong case for not so readily discarding the analytical concept of disciplines. As I have demonstrated through a concentration on the discursive identity-formation of research communities, the concept is compatible with the messier view of science that is characteristic of STS and their emphasis on research practices and cultures. However, a concentration on only the quotidian features of science fails to account for the structural relationships that transcend the micro-social and material conditions of research. Though my study revealed how the institutions of medicine have over the past roughly two-hundred and twenty years fragmented into several different ones – some with closer proximity to the everyday realities of clinical practice than others – it also showed that they are all held together by overarching narratives and ideals, such as those contained in the super-categories scientific medicine and biomedicine. In this respect, despite the different methods of research, various understandings of science and conflicting languages of practice, investigating how professional actors articulate their common identity nevertheless enables mediation between the level of the everyday realities experienced by them and the level of the larger structural context of boundaries, relationships and institutions that define the system in which they operate.

The idea of disciplinary identity was used to suggest a connection of local cultures of research with global narratives of science. The observed identity work by actors in the medical science sector, moreover, makes clear how discipline formation – strictly speaking – is a dynamic and permanent process. Actors continuously adapted the identity of their discipline to the changing settings of research policy and societal expectations. Protagonists who defined medicine's disciplinary identity all aimed at conserving or promoting a certain medical research culture. This meant securing the social, political and cultural legitimation of their research trajectories as well as facilitating recruitment into the ranks of their scientific profession. The analytical framework combining the notion of disciplinary cultures with an approach to studying discursive identity work proved rewarding in examining the disciplinary dynamics of medical science and therefore makes a fruitful addition to the social and cultural study of science. I could show how the disciplinary identity work of historical actors fulfilled the function of securing the persistence of their research trajectories and autonomous scientific pursuits by equipping their autonomous discipline with promises of utility. This ranged from the more abstract and cultural idea of providing a certain form of education but could also manifest itself in more concrete "services", such as understanding the nature of disease or contributing to health care practices. It became obvious that an adherence to overarching scientific narratives played an important role for structuring the medical discipline as well as its relation to other sciences and society more broadly.

The classification of medicine as *Wissenschaft* in early-nineteenth-century Germany, which connected it to the pure science ideal of Romanticism, for instance, first enabled the development of an autonomous discipline of medical science. As actors began refraining from practicing medicine to pursue scientific work, they could legitimize their new form of medical occupation with the argument that exposure of medical students to their science would equip them with the appropriate cognitive and moral qualities to become good physicians (and able medical scientists). Had my focus been only on the prevailing research cultures at the time, this area of occupation would have fallen to the field of what now is academic biology – which is precisely the sort of classification that many historical accounts undertake when examining these actors and their work. Similarly, had only formal structures been of interest, medicine would have become visible only as a profession and would not have been seen to emerge as a full-blown academic discipline in the modern research university.

Keeping the local circumstances and the overarching narratives of science in view, was crucial also in other instances, for example, when clinical medicine began to be framed as a pure science at the start of the twentieth century in the USA. American protagonists imported European ideals and interests of science (particularly those who had studied and worked at German institutions) and adapted them to the academic system in the United States. A view to formal structures would have only revealed the distinction between medical science and clinical medicine, on the one side, and biology and medicine on the other. Taking the pure science vocabulary into view, however, enabled a perspective on how the methods and ideals of experimental work also spread to clinical medicine. This helped understanding how under the umbrella of scientific medicine a new discipline, detached from the research practice of medical laboratory science, was beginning to form. At the same time, this transfer not only complicated the relationship of medical science and clinical practice. It also became obvious how biological and medical science research cultures moved closer together.

Biomedical science inherited its disciplinary identity from the distinction of medical science and clinical medicine as well as from the convergence of biological and medical research cultures after World War II. Contextualizing these developments in the post-war narrative of basic science helped comprehend how the previous spread of experimental work in medicine also to the natural sciences departments caused serious ambiguities with respect to their institutional affiliation and to actors' professional work. Regarding the national science policy after World War II, the adjective "biomedical" emerged as a shorthand for collectively grouping research activities in medical and biological institutions in order to correct the ambiguity. But since the concept of the life sciences already defined this large group of work with a view to methodology and subject, the primary identification of biomedical science no longer is a specific method or a clearly demarcated subject area, but instead what I have called a linear legacy – the rather remote promise that basic laboratory investigations will pay off in health care benefits in the future. However, following the crises in clinical research towards the end of the twentieth century, new concepts emerged. While EBM contains the idea of biomedicine as an independent academic discipline, TR preserves the linear legacy, which determines our overall understanding of the modern enterprise.

I have further suggested that "biomedicine" today acts as both the name for a vast academic meta-discipline *and* as an integrational supercategory. This distinction becomes apparent when we see how the label is enlisted to signify the system of research-based medicine as a whole, as opposed to only the part that frames basic laboratory research as contributing to public health care. In contrast to the discipline, therefore, which is defined by the above-mentioned distinction and convergence, the supercategory sees only integration: purely biological research with no clinical implications as well clearly clinical work have become subsumed under the label of biomedicine. This analytical perspective – name for a discipline vs. supercategory – can help us make sense of the current ambiguities and conflicts, which appear to burden the health care system. As I have shown, the actors defining, reorienting and refining the role of the scientific discipline of medicine with respect to the world of academia and the requirements of medical practice and training, simultaneously also contributed to the supercategorical function of describing the modern enterprise globally. A crucial point in this respect is to clearly spell out what distinguishes the scientific discipline from the global understanding and the social promises attached to it. To wrap up my investigation, I want to give examples that will help elucidate this analytical advantage.

The problem at hand appears to be that we cannot distinguish between the legitimate and unjustified demands that can be brought to the discipline of biomedical science. Our image of the field seems tainted by overburdened expectations in public discourses. What does biomedical science offer as viable services to medicine, other fields and society more broadly? One way to sociologically assess the roles and expectations associated with the term biomedicine is to distinguish more clearly between self-depictions of the discipline and more general narratives of science and medical progress. In the case of today's biomedicine, the discipline is not primarily characterized by its research subject, nor only by an ostensible outlook to the improvement of health care, but much more narrowly by specialized job opportunities and very concrete services to other social realms.

The Life & Medical Sciences Institute of the University of Bonn, for example, currently offers an elite three-year Bachelor's course in "Molecular

Biomedicine".[85] The curriculum is composed of general physics, chemistry and biochemistry, immunology, microbiology, genetics, developmental biology, anatomy, cell biology, neurobiology and physiology, molecular medicine, pharmacology, pathology – a classic list of subjects in the hybrid curriculum that will deliver proficiency in the research culture of biomedicine. The course's core description references the hybridity and alludes to the linear legacy, as I have explicated it:

> "The Bachelor's course in Molecular Biomedicine combines methods and the molecular understanding of the natural sciences with current contents of medicine. The goal is to obtain a molecular understanding of the mechanisms and functions of complex life processes and to understand the pathophysiology of human diseases. This is also the basis for the development of new diagnostics and therapy approaches, which are intended to combat human diseases".[86]

The discipline thus adheres to its identity of the linear legacy, asserting that its work is basic to the future improvement of public health. Moreover, the course of Molecular Biomedicine is offered at the medical faculty in Bonn and much of the training takes place in university hospital facilities. One would therefore be inclined to see the proximity to clinical medicine and hospital work. However, the description of services and job prospects removed from clinical interests confirms my thesis that biomedical science has grown into an autonomous academic discipline. Looking at the professed service roles, the discipline appears in a much humbler light. In their advertisement of the bachelor's course, the university lists the following as possible occupational fields for graduates: "basic biomedical research (institutes of the Max-Planck-Society, major research institutions etc.), development/production/marketing (industry), molecular diagnostic (for medical, biotechnical, environment-related, forensic issues; in clinical disciplines – e.g. pediatrics, human genetics, internal medicine), science (teaching/research at universities, research institutes etc.)."[87]

Consequently, next to the prospect of a traditional academic career, the subject is thus directed towards two large areas of services: one is the

---

85 See https://limes-institut-bonn.de/studium-lehre/bsc-molekulare-biomedizin/ (accessed August 17, 2020).

86 https: //limes-institut-bonn.de/en/education-training/bsc-molecular-biomedicine/ (accessed August 17, 2020).

87 https://www.uni-bonn.de/studium/vor-dem-studium/faecher/molekulare-biomed izin/molekulare-biomedizin-bachelor-of-science/molekulare-biomedizin-bachelor -of-science-ein-fach?set_language=de (accessed August 17, 2020).

employment of expertise in various settings of research and development; the other is the application to diagnostic problems. There is no explicit mention of discoveries of disease and curing the sick. Graduates of Molecular Biomedicine are neither oriented specifically towards the solution of clinical problems nor do they any longer seem necessarily responsible for medicine in a large sense. Where their work is directed to medical issues, and not to subjects like the environment or forensics, it appears that their work and training is almost directed towards those areas, which Ahrens and others felt were threatening the integrity of clinical research in the last decades of the twentieth century.

Abstracting again to the general level, this means that, although formally housed in a medical institution, the discipline developed independently from its epistemic and practical requirements. Furthermore, it becomes apparent how it is a direct descendant of the culture that emerged after 1800 and which was interested only in the pure science of organic nature. In other words, recognizing biomedical science as an autonomous discipline helps to better categorize the field into the general system of science and academia, seeing how it relates to societal expectations and to prospects for advancing science and the treatment of disease.

This analytical perspective can reveal some of the far-reaching consequences that have resulted from regarding biomedicine, in a supercategorical fashion, as the general name for the academic health care system. In 2009, Iain Chalmers and Paul Glasziou, both towering figures in EBM, for instance, published an alarming evaluation of the research-based health care system's current state in *The Lancet*. Their revelation was that large parts of research outcomes were going to waste because they proved unusable for clinical purposes. Chalmers and Glasziou identified that globally "over US$100 billion is invested every year in supporting biomedical research", which leads to "an estimated 1 million research publications" annually (2009: 86). The authors refer to biomedicine as a supercategory, and not a discipline, since they speak of how the largest part of this money goes to "basic research", with only a fraction devoted to "treatment evaluation" – their own area of expertise (ibid.). Just as became clear with other commentators, the authors are thereby implying that biomedicine comprises more than only a laboratory research culture. Nonetheless, Chalmers and Glasziou warn the academic medical community, and the public more generally, that the high investments in the academic health care system "should be protected from avoidable waste of inadequately producing and reporting research" (ibid.).[88]

Chalmers' and Galsziou's study is based mostly on data that reveals research waste coming from the conduction of and reporting on clinical trials, but they "believe it is reasonable to assume that problems also apply to other types of research", which – in accordance with the supercategorical understanding – suggests extrapolating their findings to the biomedical research system as a whole (ibid: 88). The authors identify four stages in the research process in which losses can occur: research question, research design and methods, access to publications and the usability of reported findings. Out of theses stages, therefore, two pertain to the production and two to the publication of research. The various biases plaguing scientific publication processes are an enduring theme that has been dealt with in a row of analyses in science studies (Leng/Leng 2020: 199–226). I want to confine my argument only to the first two aspects concerning knowledge production, since it is highly relevant to the issue of the relationship between science and medicine, which I have pursued in my book.

The complaints brought forth specifically by Chalmers and Glasziou concerning research production are, on the one hand, that researchers can address "the wrong questions for research" or, on the other, pursue "studies that are unnecessary, or poorly designed" (2009: 86f.). But what are the *right* questions? And how is their "correctness" determined? It must be understood that such questions are predetermined by the scientific narratives to which a discipline adheres and consequently also by the societal expectations it is connected to. Very simply, for example, it would be spurious to expect concrete outcomes from research that qualifies itself as basic research or to expect material gains or products from the social sciences and humanities (although, sadly, this seems to be the measuring stick for some research policies). For evaluations of the research process this means keeping the two dimensions in mind. Stated differently, the waste problem in biomedical research turns out to pose itself in light of specific imperatives that justify the production of scientific knowledge in front of the background of a sense of urgency: namely, the need to heal disease. With respect to the first complaint, therefore, the imperative is that an "efficient system of research should address health problems of importance to populations"; "However," Chalmers and Glasziou observe, "public funding of research is correlated only modestly with disease burden, if at all" (ibid). The second imperative concerns the pursuit of "new

---

88 Glasziou and Chalmers (2018) renewed their warning recently.

research", which the authors see only justified if, "at the time it is initiated, the question it proposes to address cannot be answered satisfactorily with existing evidence" (ibid: 87).

From a social and ethical perspective, Chalmers and Glasziou are making very reasonable demands to better understand and improve the processes of research production and reporting. Even on a modest scale, this would promise "to yield substantially increased dividends for patients and the public" (ibid.). However, they are making these demands without a clear view of the actual promises of biomedicine. The generality with which these demands are expressed reveals the confusion that exists over whether all of the different research operations bearing the name of the supercategory biomedicine actually pursue the explicit end of improving the healing of disease. I was able to show that the academic health care system is characterized by fragmentation into heterogenous research cultures with actors pursuing vastly different aims and very particular interests. In fact, many can apply the label biomedicine to describe their research work without any direct intention of improving health care. Again, my investigation revealed that the key concept of biomedicine, which is the dominant term in the present science and policy discourses, is at the same time a supercategory subsuming a variety of different activities and transporting a linear legacy that connects improvements in public health with research work; but, as biomedical science, also the name of an autonomous scientific discipline, largely removed from issues of clinical medicine. It is no trivial matter that Chalmers and Glasziou, key actors in academic medicine with a great deal of influence, fail to see – or at least clearly express – this difference in their text, since thereby their ostensibly reasonable demands, in fact, turn out to be founded on false expectations. In short, Chalmers and Glasziou seem to demand from individual research fields what only the supercategory of biomedicine promises.

More, my focus on the use of medicine's conceptual language allowed contrasting the idea of modern medicine as a discipline with our common understanding of medicine as a profession and can also open up a valuable analytical vantage point with respect to current issues. For instance, those works dealing with the historical category of scientific medicine were characterized by the sharp analytical distinction between the clinic and the laboratory, while the social and historical studies of biomedicine seem to have been constructed more from the background of how innovations in research practices have somehow also enabled better practical abilities of medicine. Both have in common, though, that they underplay the identity of medicine as a scientific discipline and inflate its understanding as a profession. In the majority of social and historical studies of medicine, the enterprise is thus presented as constituted by the application of scientific knowledge.

As a result, medicine has been conceptualized in terms of its conflicting scientific and practical identity. This biased understanding of medicine might also help explain why Chalmers and Glasziou make such generalizing demands of a highly complex and differentiated system. Regularly, questions arise to whether scientific prescriptions or the practical experience of the physician should govern clinical decision making (as in debates around EBM, for example). But if we see medicine in the light of a scientific discipline, contemporary conflicts over how much science should guide the actions of practicing physicians can be viewed more in the light of boundary disputes between proponents of medicine as science and as a profession, respectively, and about ambiguous formulations of what to expect of the discipline's services. Moreover, if we distinguish between the overall expectations attached to the supercategory, which are also reflected in our view of the profession's abilities, and the concrete services of the discipline, it will become easier to differentiate between which research outputs constitute waste and which simply address questions that do not relate to the general issue of clinical practice (notwithstanding that problems of research quality exist). This view should inspire the assessment of future research policies regarding the relationship between input and outcome and to whether the current policies might be fueling the perceived crises by investing in unrealistic expectations of what research-based medicine can and cannot do.

Bibliography

Abbott, Andrew. 2001. *Chaos of Disciplines.* Chicago/London: Chicago University Press.

Ahrens, Edward H. 1992. *The Crisis in Clinical Research. Overcoming Institutional Obstacles.* New York/Oxford: Oxford University Press.

Amsterdamska, Olga. 2005. Demarcating Epidemiology. *Science, Technology, & Human Values* 30(1) Special Issue: *Demarcation Socialized. Constructing Boundaries and Recognizing Difference*: 17–51.

Amundsen, Darrel W. 1979. Medicine and Surgery as Art or Craft. The Role of Schematic Literature in the Separation of Medicine and Surgery in the Late Middle Ages. *Transactions & Studies of the College of Physicians of Philadelphia* 1(1): 43–57.

Appel, Toby A. 1987. Biological and Medical Societies and the Founding of the American Physiological Society. *Physiology in the American Context, 1850–1940.* Ed. Gerald L. Geison. New York: Springer. 155–176.

Appel, Toby A. 1991. Organizing Biology. The American Society of Naturalists and its "Affiliated Societies", 1883–1923. *The American Development of Biology.* Ed. Ronald Rainger / Keith R. Benson / Jane Maienschein. New Brunswick/London: Rutgers University Press. 87–120.

Appel, Toby A. 2000. *Shaping Biology. The National Science Foundation and American Biological Research, 1945–1975.* Baltimore/London: Johns Hopkins University Press.

Armstrong, David. 2007. Professionalism, Indeterminacy and the EBM Project. *BioSocieties* 2(1): 73–84.

Ash, Mitchell G. 2019. Interdisciplinarity in Historical Perspective. *Perspectives on Science* 27(4): 619–642.

Barker, Lewellys F. 1908. Medical Laboratories. Their Relations to Medical Practice and Medical Discovery. *Science* 27(694): 601–611.

Barker, Lewellys F. 1913. On the Cultivation of the Clinical Sciences of Diagnosis and Therapy. *Science* 37(959): 731–738.

Barker, Lewellys F. 1916. Relation of the Preclinical Laboratory Courses to the Work of the Clinical Years. *JAMA* 66(9): 631–635.

Barnes, Barry / Bloor, David / Henry, John. 1996. *Scientific Knowledge. A Sociological Analysis.* Chicago/London: University of Chicago Press.

Becher, Tony / Trowler, Paul R. 2001. *Academic Tribes and Territories. Intellectual Enquiry and the Culture of Disciplines.* 2nd ed. Maidenhead: The Society for Research into Higher Education / Open University Press.

Benson, Keith R. 1991. From Museum Research to Laboratory Research. The Transformation of Natural History into Academic Biology. *The American Development of Biology*. Ed. Ronald Rainger / Keith R. Benson / Jane Maienschein. New Brunswick/London: Rutgers University Press. 49–83.

Berliner, Howard S. 1985. *A System of Scientific Medicine. Philanthropic Foundations in the Flexner Era*. New York/London: Travistock.

Bleker, Johanna. 1981. *Die Naturhistorische Schule, 1825–1645. Ein Beitrag zur Geschichte der klinischen Medizin in Deutschland*. Stuttgart: Fischer.

Bleker, Johanna. 1987/88. Medical Students – to the Bed-Side or to the Laboratory? The Emergence of Laboratory-Training in German Medical Education, 1870–1900. *Clio Medica* 21(1/4): 35–46.

Benaroyo, Lazare. 1998. Rudolf Virchow and the Scientific Approach to Medicine. *Endeavour* 22(3). 114–116.

Bonner, Thomas N. 1990. The German Model of Training Physicians in the United States, 1870–1914. How Closely was it Followed? *Bulletin of the History of Medicine* 64(1): 18–34.

Bonner, Thomas N. 1995a. *Becoming a Physician. Medical Education in Britain, France, Germany, and the United States, 1750–1945*. New York/Oxford: Oxford University Press.

Bonner, Thomas N. 1995b. German Influences on American Clinical Medicine, 1870–1914. *German Influences on Education in the United States to 1917*. Ed. Henry Geitz / Jürgen Heideking / Jurgen Herbst. Cambridge: Cambridge University Press. 275–287.

Borck, Cornelius. 2020. Negotiating Epistemic Hierarchies in Biomedicine: The Rise and Fall of Evidence-based Medicine. *Weak Knowledge: Forms, Functions, and Dynamics*. Ed. Moritz Epple / Annette Imhausen / Falk Müller. Frankfurt/New York: Campus. 449–482.

Bourdieu, Pierre. 1975. The Specificity of the Scientific Field and the Social Conditions of the Progress of Reason. *Social Science Information* 14(6). 19–47.

Bourdieu, Pierre. 1990. *The Logic of Practice*. Cambridge: Polity Press.

Bourdieu, Pierre / Wacquant, Loïc J.D. 1992. *An Invitation to Reflexive Sociology*. Chicago/London: University of Chicago Press.

Broman, Thomas. 1989. University Reform in Medical Thought at the End of the Eighteenth Century. *Osiris* 5: 36–53.

Broman, Thomas. 1991. J. C. Reil and the "Journalization" of Physiology. *The Literary Structure of Scientific Arguments. Historical Studies*. Ed. Peter Dear. Philadelphia: University of Pennsylvania Press.

Broman, Thomas. 1996. *The Transformation of German Academic Medicine, 1750–1820*. Cambridge: Cambridge University Press.

Bruchhausen, Walter. 2010. "Biomedizin" in sozial- und kulturwissenschaftlichen Beiträgen. Eine Begriffskariere zwischen Analyse und Polemik. *N.T.M.* 18.

Bud, Robert. 2007. *Penicillin. Triumph and Tragedy*. Oxford/New York: Oxford University Press.

Bud, Robert. 2014. Applied Science in Nineteenth-Century Britain. Public Discourse and the Creation of Meaning, 1817–1876. History and Technology 30(4): 1–34.

Bush, Vannevar. 1995 [1945]. *Science – The Endless Frontier.* North Stratford, N.H.: Ayer Company Publishers.

Butler, Declan. 2008. Translational Research. Crossing the Valley of Death. *Nature* 453: 840–842.

Bylebyl, Jerome J. 1990. The Medical Meaning of *Physica. Osiris* 6: 16–41.

Bynum; William. 1994. *Science and the Practice of Medicine in the Nineteenth Century.* Cambridge: Cambridge University Press.

Cahan, David (ed.). 2003. *From Natural Philosophy to the Sciences. Writing the History of Nineteenth-Century Science.* Chicago/London: University of Chicago Press.

Cambrosio, Alberto / Keating, Peter / Schlich, Thomas / Weisz, George. 2006. Regulatory Objectivity and the Generation and Management of Evidence in Medicine. *Social Science & Medicine* 63: 189–199.

Chadarevian, Soraya de / Kamminga, Harmke (eds.). 1998. Molecularizing Biology and Medicine. New Perspectives and Alliances, 1910s-1970s. Amsterdam: Harwood.

Chalmers, Iain / Glasziou, Paul. 2009. Avoidable Waste in the Production and Reporting of Research Evidence. *The Lancet* 374: 86–89.

Clarke, Adele E. / Shim, Janet K. / Mamo, Laura / Fosket, Jennifer Ruth / Fishman / Jennifer R. 2003. Biomedicalization. Technoscientific Transformations of Health, Illness, and US Biomedicine. *American Sociological Review* 68(2). 161–194.

Clarke, Sabine. 2010. Pure Science with a Practical Aim. The Meanings of Fundamental Research in Britain, circa 1916–1950. *Isis* 101(2): 285–311.

Cohen, Michael Aaron / Stavri, P. Zoë / Hersch, William R. 2004. A Categorization and Analysis of The Criticisms of Evidence-Based Medicine. *International Journal of Medical Informatics* 73: 35–43.

Coleman, William. 1988. Prussian Pedagogy. Purkyně at Breslau, 1823–1829. *The Investigative Enterprise. Experimental Physiology in Nineteenth-Century Medicine.* Ed. William Coleman / Frederic L. Holmes. Berkley et al.: University of California Press. 15–64.

Cooper, Joseph D. 1965. Onward the Management of Science. The Woolridge Report. *Science* 148(3676): 1433–1439.

Crabu, Stefano. 2018. Rethinking Biomedicine in the Age of Translational Research. Organizational, Professional, and Epistemic Encounters. *Sociology Compass* e12623. doi.org/10.1111/soc4.12623.

Cunningham, Andrew. 2002. The pen and the sword. Recovering the disciplinary identity of physiology and anatomy before 1800. I: Old physiology – the pen. *Studies in the History and Philosophy of Biological and Biomedical Sciences* 33: 631–665.

Cunningham, Andrew. 2003. The pen and the sword. Recovering the disciplinary identity of physiology and anatomy before 1800. II: Old anatomy – the sword. *Studies in the History and Philosophy of Biological and Biomedical Sciences* 34: 51–76.

Daly, Jeanne. 2005. *Evidence-Based Medicine and the Search for a Science of Clinical Care.* Berkley et al.: University of California Press/Milbank Memorial Fund.

Davis, Nathan S. 1891. The Basis of Scientific Medicine and the Proper Methods of Investigation. *JAMA* 16(4): 114–120.

Dewey, John. 1910. Science as Subject-Matter and as Method. *Science* 31(787): 121–127.

Dewey, John. 1997. *How We Think.* Mineola: Dover.

Evidence-Based Medicine Working Group. 1992. Evidence-based medicine. A new approach to teaching the practice of medicine. *JAMA* 268(17): 2420–2425.

Feinstein, Alvan. 1995. The Crisis in Clinical Research. Review Essay. *Bulletin of the History of Medicine* 69(2): 288–291.

Felt, Ulrike / Igelsböck, Judith / Schikowitz, Andrea / Völker, Thomas. 2013. Growing into What? The (Un-)disciplined Socialization of Early Stage Researchers into Transdisciplinary Research. *Higher Education* 65(4): 511–524.

Felt, Ulrike / Fouché, Rayvon / Miller, Clark A. / Smith-Doerr, Laurel (eds.). 2017. *Handbook of Science and Technology Studies.* 4th ed. Cambridge, MA/London: MIT Press.

Flexner, Abraham. 1910. *Medical Education in the United States and Canada. A Report to the Carnegie Foundation for the Advancement of Teaching.* New York.

Foucault, Michel. 1973. *The Birth of the Clinic. An Archeology of Medical Perception.* Trans. A. M. Sheridan. New York: Routledge.

French, Roger, 2003. *Medicine Before Science.* Cambridge: Cambridge University Press.

Frevert, Ute. 1984. *Krankheit als politisches Problem, 1770–1880. Soziale Unterschichten in Preußen zwischen medizinischer Polizei und staatlicher Sozialversicherung.* Göttingen: Vandenhoeck & Ruprecht.

Funtowicz, Silvio O. / Ravetz, Jerome R. 1993. The Emergence of Post-Normal Science. *Science, Politics and Morality. Scientific Uncertainty and Decision-Making.* Ed. René von Schomberg. Dodrecht et al.: Kluwer. 85–123.

Fye, Bruce. 1987. *The Development of American Physiology. Scientific Medicine in the Nineteenth Century.* Baltimore/London: Johns Hopkins University Press.

Galison, Peter / Stump, David J. (eds.). 1996. *The Disunity of Science. Boundaries, Contexts, and Power.* Stanford: Stanford University Press.

Geertz, Clifford. 1983. *Local Knowledge. Further Essays in Interpretive Anthropology.* New York: Basic Books.

Geison, Gerald. 1979. Divided We Stand. Physiologists and Clinicians in the American Context. *The Therapeutic Revolution. Essays in the Social History of American Medicine.* Ed. Morris J. Vogel / Charles E. Rosenberg. Philadelphia: University of Pennsylvania Press. 67–90.

Glasziou, Paul / Chalmers, Iain. 2018. Research Wast is Still a Scandal. *BMJ* 363: k4645.

Gibbons, Michael / Limoges, Camille / Nowotny, Helga / Schwartzman, Simon / Scott, Peter / Trow, Martin. 1994. *The New Production of Knowledge. The Dynamics of Science and Research in Contemporary Societies*. Los Angeles et al.: Sage.

Gieryn, Thomas F. 1995. Boundaries of Science. *Handbook of Science and Technology Studies*. Ed. Sheila Jasanoff / Gerald E. Markle / James C. Petersen / Trevor Pinch. Rev. e ed. Thousand Oaks et al: Sage. 393–443

Gieryn, Thomas F. 1999. *Cultural Boundaries of Science. Credibility on the Line.* Chicago/London: University of Chicago Press.

Godin, Benoît. 2006. The Linear Model of Innovation. The Historical Construction of an Analytical Framework. *Science, Technology, & Human Values* 31(6). 639–667.

Godin, Benoît. 2017. *Models of Innovation. The History of an Idea.* Cambridge, MA: MIT Press.

Greenhalgh, Susan. 2008. *Just One Child. Science and Policy in Deng's China.* Berkley/Los Angeles: University of California Press.

Hackett, Edward J. / Parker, John N. / Vermeulen, Niki / Penders, Bart. 2017. The Social and Epistemic Organization of Scientific Work. *Handbook of Science and Technology Studies*. 4th ed. Ed. Ulrike Felt, and Ulrike / Fouché, Rayvon / Miller, Clark A. / Smith-Doerr, Laurel. Cambridge, MA/London: MIT Press. 733–764.

Hacking, Ian. 1992. The Self-Vindication of the Laboratory Sciences. *Science and Practice and Culture*. Ed. Andrew Pickering. Chicago/London: University of Chicago Press. 29–64.

Hacking, Ian. 2012. Introductory Essay. *The Structure of Scientific Revolutions* (Kuhn 2012). 4th ed. Chicago/London: University of Chicago Press. vii–xxxviii.

Hagner, Michael. 2003. Scientific Medicine. *From Natural Philosophy to the Sciences. Writing History of Nineteenth-Century Science*. Ed. David Cahan. Chicago/London: University of Chicago Press. 49–87.

Harris, Henry. 1999. *The Birth of the Cell*. New Haven/London: Yale University Press.

Harris, Roy. 2005. *The Semantics of Science*. London/New York: Continuum.

Harvey, A. McGhehee. 1981. *Science at the Bedside. Clinical Research in American Medicine, 1905–1945.* Baltimore/London: Johns Hopkins University Press.

Heinig, Stephen J. / Quon, Andrew S. W. / Meyer, Roger E. / Korn, David. 1999. The Changing Landscape of Clinical Research. *Academic Medicine* 74(6): 726–745.

Heller, Robert. 1975. Johann Christian Reil's Training Scheme for Medical Auxiliaries. *Medical History* 19(4): 321–332.

Hendriks, Barbara / Simons, Arno / Reinhart, Martin. 2019. What are Clinician-Scientists Expected to Do? The Undefined Space of Professionalizable Work in Translational Biomedicine. *Minerva* 57: 219–237.

Henle, Jacob. 1844. Medizinische Wissenschaft und Empirie. *Zeitschrift für rationelle Medizin* 1: 1–35.

Hess, Volker. 1993. *Von der semiotischen zur diagnostischen Medizin. Die Entstehung der klinischen Methode zwischen 1750 und 1850.* Husum: Matthisen.

Hess, Volker. 1994. Objektivität und Rhetorik. Karl August Wunderlich (1815–1877) und die klinische Thermometrie. *Medizinhistorisches Journal* 32(3/4). 299–319.

Hess, Volker. 1995. Diagnose und Krankheitsverständnis der medizinischen Klinik der Berliner Universität, 1820–1845. *Abhandlungen zur Geschichte der Medizin und Naturwissenschaften* 67: 101–10.

Hess, Volker. 2010a. Die Alte Charité, die moderne Irrenabteilung und die Klinik (1790–1820). *Die Charité. Geschichte(n) eines Krankenhauses.* Ed. Johanna Bleker / Volker Hess. Berlin Akademie Verlag. 44–69.

Volker Hess. 2010b. Fieberbehandlung und klinische Wissenschaft (1820–1850). *Die Charité. Geschichte(n) eines Krankenhauses.* Ed. Johanna Bleker / Volker Hess. Berlin Akademie Verlag. 70–98.

Hippocrates. 2012. *On the Art of Medicine.* Ed., trans., & commentary Joel E. Mann. Leiden/Boston: Brill.

Höpfner, Ludwig Julius Friedrich, 1778. *Deutsche Encyclopädie oder Allgemeines Real-Wörterbuch aller Künste und Wissenschaften.* Vol. 1: A–Ar. Frankfurt/Main: Varrentrap und Wenner.

Huerkamp, Claudia. 1985. *Aufstieg der Ärzte. Vom Gelehrten Stand zum professionellen Experten. Das Beispiel Preußens.* Göttingen: Vandenhoeck & Ruprecht.

von Humboldt, Wilhelm. 1964. Über die Organisation des Medizinalwesens. *Schriften zur Politik und zum Bildungswesen (Werke in Fünf Bänden IV).* Darmstadt: Wissenschaftliche Buchgesellschaft. 56–63.

Jacobs, Jerry A. 2013. *In Defense of Disciplines. Interdisciplinarity and Specialization in the Research University.* Chicago/London: University of Chicago Press.

Jasanoff, Sheila (ed.). 2004. *States of Knowledge. The Co-Production of Science and Social Order.* London/New York: Routledge.

Jasanoff, Sheila / Kim, Sang-Hyun (eds.). 2015. *Dreamscapes of Modernity. Sociotechnical Imaginaries and the Fabrication of Power.* Chicago/London: University of Chicago Press.

Kaldewey, David. 2013. *Wahrheit und Nützlichkeit. Selbstbeschreibungen der Wissenschaft zwischen Autonomie und gesellschaftlicher Relevanz.* Bielefeld: transcript.

Kaldewey, David. 2018: The Grand Challenges Discourse. Transforming Identity Work in Science and Science Policy. *Minerva* 56: 161–182.

Kaldewey, David / Schauz, Désirée (eds.). 2018. *Basic and Applied Research. The Language of Science Policy in the Twentieth Century.* New York/Oxford: Berghahn.

Kaldewey, David / Schauz, Désirée. 2018. Transforming Pure Science into Basic Research. The Language of Science Policy in the United States. *Basic and Applied Research. The Language of Science Policy in the Twentieth Century.* Ed. David Kaldewey / Désirée Schauz. New York/Oxford: Berghahn. 104–140.

Kay, Lilly, 1993. The Molecular Vision of Life. Caltech, The Rockefeller Foundation, and the Rise of the New Biology. New York/Oxford: Oxford University Press.

Keating, Peter / Cambrosio, Alberto. 2003. *Biomedical Platforms. Realigning the normal and the pathological in late-twentieth-century medicine.* Cambridge, MA/London: MIT Press.

Keating, Peter / Cambrosio, Alberto. 2004. Does biomedicine entail the successful reduction of pathology to biology? *Perspectives in Biology and Medicine* 47(3): 357–371.

Keating, Peter / Cambrosio, Alberto. 2012. *Cancer on Trial. Oncology as a New Style of Practice.* Chicago/London: University of Chicago Press.

Knaapen, Loes. 2014. Evidence-based Medicine or Cookbook Medicine? Addressing Concerns over the Standardization of Care. *Sociology Compass* 8(6): 823–836.

Knorr Cetina, Karin / Reichmann, Werner. 2015. Art. "Epistemic Cultures." *International Encyclopedia of the Social & Behavioral Sciences.* Ed. James D. Wright. Second Ed. Vol. 7. Amsterdam: Elsevier. 873–880.

Knorr Cetina, Karin. 1981. *The Manufacture of Knowledge. An Essay on the Constructivist and Contextual Nature of Science.* Oxford et al.: Pergamon Press.

Knorr Cetina, Karin. 1999. *Epistemic Cultures. How the Sciences Make Knowledge.* Cambridge/Londong: Harvard University Press.

Kohler, Robert E. 1979. From *Medical Chemistry to Biochemistry. The Making of a Biomedical Discipline.* Cambridge: Cambridge University Press.

Kohler, Robert E. 1982. Medical Reform and Biomedical Science. Biochemistry – A Case Study. *The Therapeutic Revolution. Essays in the Social History of American Medicine.* Ed. Morris J. Vogel / Charles E. Rosenberg. Philadelphia: University of Pennsylvania Press. 27–66.

Kohler, Robert E. 1991. *Partners in Science. Foundations and Natural Scientists, 1900–1945.* Chicago/London: University of Chicago Press.

Koselleck, Reinhart. 1979. *Vergangene Zukunft. Zur Semantik geschichtlicher Zeiten.* Frankfurt: Suhrkamp.

Koselleck, Reinhart. 2006. *Begriffsgeschichten. Studien zur Semantik und Pragmatik der politischen und sozialen Sprache.* Frankfurt: Suhrkamp.

Kraft, Alison. 2013. New Light Through an Old Window? The "Translational Turn" in Biomedical Research. A Historical Perspective. *Translational Medicine. The Future of Therapy?* Ed. James Mittra / Christopher-Paul Milne. Boca Raton: CRC Press. 19–53.

Kremer, Richard L. 2009. Physiology. *The Cambridge History of Science. Volume 6: The Modern Biological and Earth Sciences.* Ed. Peter J. Bowler / John V. Pickstone. Cambridge: Cambridge University Press. 342–366.

Kuhn, Thomas S. 2012. *The Structure of Scientific Revolutions.* 4th ed. Chicago/London: University of Chicago Press.

Latour, Bruno. 1987. *Science in Action. How to Follow Scientists and Engineers Through Society.* Cambridge: Harvard University Press.

Latour, Bruno. 1998. From the World of Science to the World of Research? *Science* 280: 208–209.

Latour, Bruno / Woolgar, Steve. 1986. *Laboratory Life. The Construction of Scientific Facts*. Princeton: Princeton University Press.

Lawrence, Christopher. 1985. Incommunicable Knowledge. Science, Technology, and the Clinical Art in Britain, 1850–1914. *Journal of Contemporary History* 20(4): 503–520.

Leng, Gareth / Leng, Rhodri Ivor. 2020. *The Matter of Facts. Skepticism, Persuasion, and Evidence in Science*. Cambridge/London: MIT Press.

Lenoir, Timothy. 1997. *Instituting Science. The Cultural Production of Scientific Disciplines*. Stanford: Stanford University Press.

Lindemann, Mary. 1996. *Healing & Health in Eighteenth Century Germany*. Baltimore/London: Johns Hopkins University Press.

Lohff, Brigitte. 1981. Johannes Müllers "Jahresberichte zur Physiologie" in Müllers Archiv der Jahre 1834–1838. *Sudhoffs Archiv* 65(1): 32–78.

Löwy, Ilana. 2011. Historiography of Biomedicine. "Bio", "Medicine", and In Between. *Isis* 102(1): 116–122.

Löwy, Ilana. 1996. *Between Bench and Bedside. Science, Healing, and Interlukin-2 in a Cancer Ward*. Cambridge, MA: Harvard University Press.

Ludmerer, Kenneth M. 1996. *Learning to Heal. The Development of American Medical Education*. Baltimore/Londong: Johns Hopkins University Press.

Marks, Howard M. 1997. *The Progress of Experiment. Science and Therapeutic Reform in the United States, 1900–1990*. Cambridge: Cambridge University Press.

Mattingly, Paul H. 2017. *American Academic Cultures. A History of Higher Education*. Chicago/London: University of Chicago Press.

Maulitz, Russel C. 1978. Rudolf Virchow, Julius Cohnheim and the Program of Pathology. *Bulletin of the History of Medicine* 52. 162–182.

Maulitz, Russel C. 1979. "Physician versus Bacteriologist." The Ideology of Science in Clinical Medicine. *The Therapeutic Revolution. Essays in the Social History of American Medicine*. Ed. Morris J. Vogel / Charles E. Rosenberg. Philadelphia: University of Pennsylvania Press. 91–107.

McClelland, Charles E. 1980. *State, Society, and University in Germany 1700–1914*. Cambridge: Cambridge University Press.

McClelland, Charles E. 2013. The German Model for American medical Reform. *Themenportal Europäische Geschichte*. www.europa.clio-online.de/essay/id/fdae-15 94, accessed: 5. August 2020.

Meltzer, Samuel J. 1909. The Science of Clinical Medicine. What It Ought to Be and the Men to Uphold It. *JAMA* 53(7): 508–512.

Mittra, James. 2016. *The New Health Bioeconomy. R&D Policy and Innovation for the Twenty-First Century*. Basingstoke: Palgrave Macmillan.

Mittra, James / Milne, Christopher-Paul (eds.). 2013. *Translational Medicine. The Future of Therapy?* Boca Raton: CRC Press.

Müller, Johannes. 1834. Jahresbericht über die Fortschritte der anatomisch-physiologischen Wissenschaft im Jahre 1833. *Archiv für Anatomie, Physiologie und wissenschaftliche Medicin* 1: 1–79.

Müller, Ernst / Schmieder, Falko. 2016. *Begriffsgeschichte und historische Semantik. Ein kritisches Kompendium.* Frankfurt/Main: Suhrkamp.

NIH Study Committee [Chairman: Dean E. Wooldrige]. 1965. *Biomedical Science and its Political Administration. A Study of the National Institutes of Health.* Washington, D.C. The White House.

Nowotny, Helga / Scott, Peter / Gibbons, Michael. 2001. *Re-Thinking Science. Knowledge and the Public in an Age of Uncertainty.* Oxford: Polity.

Nyhart, Lynn K. 1995. Biology Takes Form. Animal Morphology and the German Universities, 1800–1900. Chicago/London: University of Chicago Press.

Olesko, Kathryn M. 1988. Commentary. On Institutes Investigations, and Scientific Training. *Investigative Enterprise. Experimental Physiology in Nineteenth-Century Medicine.* Ed. William Coleman / Frederic L. Holmes. Berkley et al.: University of California Press. 295–332.

Otis, Laura. 2007. *Müller's Lab.* Oxford/New York: Oxford University Press.

Pauly, Philip J. 1984. The Appearance of Academic Biology in Late Nineteenth-Century America. *Journal of the History of Biology* 17(3): 369–397.

Pauly, Philip J. 1987. General Physiology and the Discipline of Physiology, 1890–1935. *Physiology in the American Context, 1850–1940.* Ed. Gerald L. Geison. New York: Springer. 195–207.

Park, Buhm Soon. 2008. Disease Categories and Scientific Disciplines. Reorganizing the NIH Intramural Program, 1945–1960. *Biomedicine in the Twentieth Century. Practices, Policies, and Politics.* Ed. Caroline Hannaway. Amsterdam et al.: IOS Press.

Pestre, Dominique. 2003. Regimes of Knowledge Production in Society. Towards a More Political and Social Reading. *Minerva* 41(3): 245–261.

Pickstone, John V. 2000. *Ways of Knowing. A New History of Science, Technology and Medicine.* Manchester: Manchester University Press.

Phillips, Denise. 2012. *Acolytes of Nature. Defining Natural Science in Germany 1770–1850.* Chicago/London: University of Chicago Press.

Phillip, Denise. 2015. Francis Bacon and the Germans. Stories from When 'science' meant '*Wissenschaft*'. *History of Science* 53(4): 378–394.

Pickering, Andrew (ed.). 1992. *Science as Practice and Culture.* Chicago/London: University of Chicago Press.

Prüll, Cay-Rüdiger. 2000. Zwischen Krankenversorgung und Forschungsprimat. Die Pathologie

Quirke, Vivienne / Gaudillière, Jean-Paul. 2008. The Era of Biomedicine. Science, medicine and public health in Britain and France after the Second World War. *Medical History* 52: 441–452.

Rabier, Christelle. 2018. Medicalizing the Surgical Trade, 1650–1820. Workers, Knowledge, Markets and Politics. *The Palgrave Handbook of the History of Surgery.* Ed. Thomas Schlich. London: Palgrave Macmillan. 71–94.

Rasmussen, Nicolas. 2018. Biomedicine and Its Historiography. A Systematic Review. *Handbook of the History of Biology.* Ed. Michael Dietrich / Mark Borrello / Oren Harman. Cham: Springer Nature.

Reil, Johann Christian. 1804. *Pepinieren zum Unterricht ärztlicher Routiniers als Bedürfnisse des Staats nach seiner Lage wie sie ist.* Halle/Saale: Curtsche Buchhandlung.

Reil, Johann Christian. 1910. Entwurf zur Organisation einer wissenschaftlich-medizinischen Schule. *Geschichte der königlichen Friedrich-Wilhelmsuniversität zu Berlin.* Ed. Max Lenz. Vol. 3. Halle/Saale: Verlag der Buchhandlung des Waisenhauses.

Reiser, Stanley Joel. 1979. *Medicine and the Reign of Technology.* Cambridge: Cambridge University Press.

Rheinberger, Hans-Jörg. 1997. *Towards A History of Epistemic Things. Synthesizing Proteins in the Test Tube.* Stanford: Stanford University Press.

Rheinberger, Hans-Jörg. 2009. Recent Science and its Exploration: The Case of Molecular Biology. *Studies in the History and Philosophy of Biological and Biomedical Sciences* 40: 6–12.

Rosenberg, Charles E. 1997. *No Other Gods. On Science and American Social Thought.* 2. ed. Baltimore/London: Johns Hopkins University Press.

Roser, Wilhelm / Wunderlich, Karl. 1841. *Ueber die Mängel der heutigen deutschen Medicin. Programm einer neuen medicinischen Zeitschrift.* Stuttgart: Ebner & Seubert.

Roser, Wilhelm / Wunderlich, Karl. 1843. *Ueber die jetzige Lage der physiologischen Medizin.* Archiv für Physiologische Heilkunde 2: 1–5.

Roth, Phillip H. 2022. Disziplinen und Kulturen der Wissenschaft. *Wissenschaftsforschung. Grundbegriffe, Forschungsfelder und Forschungsfragen (Sozialwissenschaftliche Einführungen* 4). Ed. David Kaldewey. Berlin/Boston: De Gruyter Oldenbourg (forthcoming).

Sackett, David L. / Rosenberg, William M.C. / Gray, J. A. Muir / Haynes, R. Brian / Richardson, W. Scott. 1996. Evidence Based Medicine. What it Is and What it Isn't. *BMJ* 312: 71–72.

Schaffer, Simon. 1990. Genius in Romantic Natural Philosophy. *Romanticism and the Sciences.* Ed. Andrew Cunningham / Nicholas Jardine. Cambridge: Cambrdige University Press. 82–100-

Schatzberg, Eric. 2018. *Technology. Critical History of a Concept.* Chicago/London: Chicago.

Schauz, Désirée. 2014. What is Basic Research? Insights from Historical Semantics. *Minerva* 52(3): 273–328.

Schauz, Désirée. 2015. Wissenschaftsgeschichte und das Revival der Begriffsgeschichte. *N.T.M.* 22(3): 53–63.

Schauz, Désirée. 2020. *Nützlichkeit und Erkenntnisfortschritt. Eine Geschichte des modernen Wissenschaftsverständnisses (Deutsches Museum, Abhandlungen und Berichte 33).* Göttingen: Wallstein.

Schauz, Désirée / Kaldewey, David. 2018. Why Do Concepts Matter to Science Policy? *Basic and Applied Research. The Language of Science Policy in the Twentieth Century.* Ed. David Kaldewey / Désirée Schauz. 2018. New York/Oxford: Berghahn. 1–32.

Schauz, Désirée / Lax, Gregor. 2018. Professional Devotion, National Needs, Fascist Claims, and Democratic Values. The Language of Science Policy in Germany. *Basic and Applied Research. The Language of Science Policy in the Twentieth Century.* Ed. David Kaldewey / Désirée Schauz. 2018. New York/Oxford: Berghahn. 104–140.

Schechter, Alan N. / Perlman, Robert / Rettig, Richard A. 2004. Editor's Introduction. Why is Revitilizing Clinical Research Is So Important, Yet So Difficult? *Perspectives in Biology and Medicine* 47(4): 476–486.

Scheffler, Robin W. / Strasser, Bruno J. 2015. Art. "Biomedical Sciences, History and Sociology of." *International Encyclopedia of the Social & Behavioral Sciences.* Ed. James D. Wright. Second Ed. Vol. 2. Amsterdam: Elsevier. 663–669.

Schelling, Friedrich Wilhelm Joseph. 1974. *Vorlesungen über die Methode des akademischen Studiums.* Hamburg: Meiner.

Schelling, Friedrich Wilhelm Joseph / Marcus, Friedrich Adalbert (eds.). 1805–08. *Jahrbücher der Medicin als Wissenschaft.* Tübingen.

Schelsky, Helmut. 1971. *Einsamkeit und Freiheit. Idee und Gestalt der deutschen Universität und ihre Reform.* 2. ed. Reinbeck: Rowohlt.

Schmiedebach, Heinz-Peter. 1992. "Ist nicht wirklich diese ganze zersetzende Naturwissenschaft ein Irrweg?" Virchow und die Zellularpathologie. *Medizinhistorisches Journal* 27(1/2): 26–42.

Schneider, William H. 2015. The Origin of the Medical Research Grant in the United States. The Rockefeller Foundation and the NIH Extramural Funding Program. *Journal of the History of Medicine and Allied Sciences* 70(2): 279–311.

Schönlein, Johannes. 1926. Rede zur Eröffnung der medizinischen Klinik in Würzburg. *Deutsche Ärzte-Reden aus dem 19. Jahrhundert.* Ed. Erich Ebstein. Berlin: Springer, 6–12.

Schweber, Libby. 2006. *Disciplining Statistics. Demography and Vital Statistics in France and England, 1830–1885.* Durham/London: Duke University Press.

Shapin, Steven. 1992. Discipline and Bounding. The History and Sociology of Science as Seen Through the Externalism-Internalism Debate. *History of Science* 30: 333–369.

Shapin, Steven. 2008. *The Scientific Life. A Moral History of a Late Modern Vocation.* Chicago: University of Chicago Press.

Shapin, Steven. 2012. *Never Pure. Historical Studies of Science as If It Was Produced by People with Bodies, Situated in Time, Space, Culture, and Society, and Struggling for Credibility and Authority.* Baltimore/London: Johns Hopkins University Press.

Shinn, Terry. 2002. The Triple Helix and New Production of Knowledge. Prepackaged Thinking on Science and Technology. *Social Studies of Science* 32(4): 599–614.

Solomon, Miriam. 2011. Just a Paradigm. Evidence-Based Medicine in Epistemological Context. *European Journal of Philosophy of Science* 1(3): 451–466.

Star, Susan Leigh / Griesmer, James R. 1989. Institutional Ecology, 'Translations' and Boundary Objects. Amateurs and Professionals in Berkley's Museum of Vertebrate Zoology, 1907–39. *Social Studies of Science* 19(3): 387–420.

Starr, Paul. 1982. *The Social Transformation of American Medicine. The Rise of a Sovereign Profession and the Making of a Vast Industry.* New York: Basic Books.

Steelman, John R. 1947. *The Nation's Medical Research. A Report to the President.* Washington, D.C.: US Government Printing Office.

Stichweh, Rudolf. 1984. *Zur Entstehung des modernen Systems wissenschaftlicher Disziplinen. Physik in Deutschland, 1740–1890.* Frankfurt a.M.: Suhrkamp.

Stichweh, Rudolf. 1992. The Sociology of Scientific Disciplines. On the Genesis and Stability of the Disciplinary Structure of Modern Science. *Science in Context* 5(1): 3–15.

Stichweh, Rudolf. 1994a. Professionen und Disziplinen. Formen der Differenzierung zweier Systeme beruflichen Handelns in modernen Gesellschaften. *Wissenschaft, Universität, Profession. Soziologische Analysen.* Frankfurt/Main: Suhrkamp. 278–336.

Stichweh, Rudolf. 1994b. The Unity of Teaching and Research. *Romanticism in the Science. Science in Europe, 1780–1840.* Ed. Stefano Poggi / Maurizio Bossi. Dodrecht/Boston: Kluwer. 189–202.

Stichweh, Rudolf. 2007. Einheit und Differenz im Wissenschaftssystem der Moderne. *Zwei Kulturen der Wissenschaft – revisited.* Ed. Jost Halfmann / Johannes Rohbeck. Weilerswits: Velbrück Wissenschaft. 213–228.

Strasser, Bruno. 2014. *Biomedicine. Meanings, assumptions, and possible futures.* Report to the Swiss Science and Innovation Council.

Sturdy, Steve. 2011. Looking for Trouble. Medical Science and Clinical Practice in the Historiography of Modern Medicine. *Social History of Medicine* 24(3): 739–757.

Swain, Donald C. 1962. The Rise of a Research Empire. NIH, 1930 to 1950. *Science* 138(3546): 1233–1237.

Timmermans, Stefan / Berg, Marc. 2003. *The Gold Standard. The Challenge of Evidence-Based Medicine and Standardization of Health Care.* Philadelphia: Temple University Press.

Timmermans, Stefan / Kolker, Emily S. 2004. Evidence-Based Medicine and the Reconfiguration of Medical Knowledge. *Journal of Health and Social Behavior* 45: 177–193.

Trowler, Paul. 2014. Academic Tribes and Territories. The Theoretical Trajectory. *Österreichische Zeitschrift für Geschichtswissenschaften* 25(3). 17–26.

Tuchman, Arleen Marcia. 1993. *Science, Medicine, and the State in Germany. The Case of Baden, 1815–1871.* Oxford: Oxford University Press.

Tuchman, Arleen. 2000. Ein verwirrendes Dreieck. Universität, Charité, Pépinière. *Jahrbuch für Universitätsgeschichte* 3: 36–47.

Turner, Stephen. 2000. What are Disciplines? And How is Interdisciplinarity Different? Interdisciplinarity. The Paradoxical Discourse. *Practicing Interdisciplinarity.* Ed. Perter Weingart / Nico Stehr. Toronto et al.: University of Toronto Press. 46–65.

Turner, Stephen. 2017. Knowledge Formations. An Analytic Framework. *The Oxford Handbook of Interdisciplinarity.* 2nd ed. Ed. Robert Frodeman / Julie Thompson Klein / Roberto C. S. Pacheco. Oxford: Oxford University Press. 9–20.

Turner, Steven R. 1980. *Bildungsbürgertum* and the Learned Professions in Prussia, 1770–1830. The Origins of a Class. *Histoire Sociale Social History* 12(25): 105–135.

US Senate, Committee on Government Operations. 1959. *The National Science Foundation and the Life Sciences.* Washington, D.C.

Van der Laan, Anna Laura / Boenink, Marianne. 2015. Beyond Bench and Bedside. Disentangling the Concept of Translational Research. *Health Care Analysis* 23: 32–49.

Vignola-Gagné, Etienne. 2014. Argumentative Practices in Science, Technology and Innovation Policy. The Case of Clinician-Scientists and Translational Research. *Science and Public Policy* 41: 94–106.

Virchow, Rudolf. 1847. Ueber die Standpunkte in der wissenschaftlichen Medicin. *Archiv für pathologische Anatomie, Physiologie und klinische Medicin* 1: 3–19.

Virchow, Rudolf. 1849. Die naturwissenschaftliche Methode und die Standpunkte in der Therapie. *Archiv für pathologische Anatomie, Physiologie und klinische Medicin* 2: 3–37.

Virchow, Rudolf. 1855. Cellular-Pathologie. *Archiv für pathologische Anatomie, Physiologie und klinische Medicin* 8: 3–39.

Virchow, Rudolf. 1877. Ueber die Standpunkte in der wissenschaftlichen Medicin. *Archiv für pathologische Anatomie, Physiologie und klinische Medicin* 70(1): 1–10.

Virchow, Rudolf. 1958. *Disease, Life, and Man. Selected Essays by Rudolf Virchow.* Trans. Lelland J. Rather. Stanford: Stanford University Press.

Vogd, Werner. 2002. Professionalisierungsschub oder Auflösung ärztlicher Autonomie? Die Bedeutung von Evidence Based Medicine und der neuen Funktionalen Eliten in der Medizin aus system- und interaktionstheoretischer Perspektive. *Zeitschrift für Soziologie* 31(4): 294–315.

Waddington, Ivan. 1990. The Movement Towards the Professionalization of Medicine. *BMJ* 301: 688–690.

Wallis, Faith. 2018. Pre-Modern Surgery. Wounds, Words, and the Paradox of "Tradition". *The Palgrave Handbook of the History of Surgery.* Ed. Thomas Schlich. London: Palgrave Macmillan. 49–70.

Warner, John Harley. 1985. Science in Medicine. *Osiris* 1: 37–58.

Warner, John Harley. 1986. *The Therapeutic Perspective. Medical Practice, Knowledge, and Identity in America, 1820–1885.* Cambridge, M.A./London: Harvard University Press.

Warner, John Harley. 1991. Ideals of Science and their Discontents in Late Nineteenth-Century American Medicine. *Isis* 82(3): 454–478.

Warner, John Harley. 1992. The Rise and Fall of Professional Mystery. Epistemology, authority and the emergence of laboratory medicine in nineteenth-century America. *The Laboratory Revolution in Medicine*. Ed. Andrew Cunningham / Perry Williams. Cambridge: Cambridge University Press. 110–141.

Warner, John Harley. 1995. The History of Science and the Sciences of Medicine. *Osiris* 10: 164–193.

Weingart, Peter. 2000. Interdisciplinarity. The Paradoxical Discourse. *Practicing Interdisciplinarity*. Ed. Perter Weingart / Nico Stehr. Toronto et al.: University of Toronto Press. 25–41.

Weingart, Peter. 2010. A Short History of Knowledge Formations. *The Oxford Handbook of Interdisciplinarity*. Ed. Julie Thompson Klein / Carl Mitcham. Oxford/New York: Oxford University Press. 3–14.

Weisz, George. 2005. From Clinical Counting to Evidence-Based Medicine. *Body Counts. Medical Quantification in Historical & Sociological Perspective*. Ed. Gérard Jorland / Annick Opinel / George Weisz. Montreal et al.: McGill-Queen's University Press. 377–393.

Weisz, George. 2006. *Divide and Conquer. A Comparative History of Medical Specialization*. Oxford/New York: Oxford University Press.

Weisz, George / Cambrosio, Alberto / Keating, Peter / Knaapen, Loes / Schlich, Thomas / Tournay, Virginie J. 2007. The Emergence of Clinical Practice Guidelines. *The Milbank Quarterly* 85(4): 691–727.

Wimmer, Mario. 2015. "Conceptual History: Begriffsgeschichte." *International Encyclopedia of the Social & Behavioral Sciences*. Ed. James D. Wright. Second Ed. Vol. 2. Amsterdam: Elsevier. 548–554.

Wilson-Kovacz, Dana / Hauskeller, Christine. 2012. The Clinician-Scientist. Professional Dynamics in Clinical Stem Cell Research. *Sociology of Health & Illness* 34(4): 497–512.

Wunderlich, Karl. 1845. Das Verhältniss der physiologischen Medicin zur ärztlichen Praxis. *Archiv für physiologische Heilkunde* 4. 1–13.

Zammito, John. 2018. *The Gestation of German Biology. Physiology and Philosophy from Stahl to Schelling*. Chicago/London: University of Chicago Press.

Zerhouni, Elias. 2003. The NIH Roadmap. *Science* 302: 63–72.